How To Make It In Nursing As A Man

How To Thrive, Persevere, And Become A Success In Your Journey To Earning The Title Of A Male Nurse

Patrice M Foster

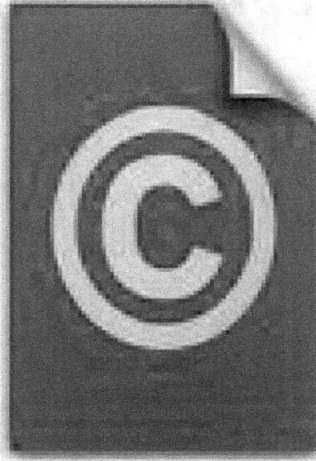

Table of Contents

Introduction

Entering the medical field requires a specific type of personality. Hard work, perseverance, determination, and selflessness are but a few of the most prominent qualities that anyone in the medical field needs to possess.

However, becoming a male nurse takes all of that and more. Having picked up this book, you are either an already qualified male nurse or want to apply to become one.

At this point, it is essential to mention that becoming a male nurse takes guts. You are entering a predominantly female profession. But, you are playing a pivotal role many women nurses cannot fulfill. Just imagine a male patient that needs to be washed and cared for at the bedside. Many may feel uncomfortable having a female nurse assisting them on their journey to recovery. This is exactly where the role of becoming a male nurse fits in!

A male nurse balances out the nursing profession. They may get a lot of backlash for wanting to break the gender stereotype associated with the nursing profession. However, you cannot deny your calling, especially if it is one where placing others before yourself, caring for them in their end stages of life, as well as providing them a foundation of perfect health for them to achieve success is always at the forefront of your mind.

Edward Lyon, Joe Hogan, Walt Whitman, and Luther Christman are some famous names that have already started to break the stereotype of a woman-only nursing profession. They have not only found a home within the nursing profession but, contrastingly, have faced strife and discrimination for wanting to be male nurses. Their sheer determination to stick with their passion and calling led Luther Christman to form the National Male Nursing Association (NMNA). These change agents have paved the way for you, too, to enter into the nursing profession without any form of shame!

In this book, we will discuss the journey of the male nurse. This includes the initial thoughts that you may have about wanting to become a male nurse, the process that you will need to follow, and the benefits of being a male nurse, as well as debunking some myths that individuals may have about male nurses.

This book is more than just about becoming a male nurse; it is about becoming part of a team of healthcare professionals who care for patients and allow them to get back to their most optimal level of functioning. With that, there will most likely be a few coworker issues that may arise. Some individuals may struggle to be able to separate their professional life from their personal life. This can result in conflict within the workplace. This is normal, but it needs a specific approach if you are going to ensure that it doesn't get in the way of providing the best care to your patients.

You will inevitably interact with healthcare professionals who have veered away from focusing on the care provided to their patients and more on how they can make more money. But, how you approach these professionals will dictate the degree of success that you will have in establishing meaningful interpersonal relationships in the workplace. Don't worry; we will be tackling all of this a bit later in this book.

You were meant to be a male nurse, and we will teach you how to not only become a male nurse but also thrive, persevere, and succeed!

Chapter 1: How to Introduce the Nursing Profession to Teenage Boys

The thought of becoming a male nurse has definitely crossed the minds of many teenage boys. However, they have either been persuaded otherwise by the people around them or have been led to believe that the nursing profession is only for women.

So, how do we change this mindset and introduce teenage boys to the possibility of becoming male nurses?

One of the main points of resistance that teenage boys face is that it isn't 'manly' enough. This has everything to do with perception! Nursing, in general, requires quick thinking, high levels of stamina, and a certain degree of physical strength.

Does this not perfectly fit one of the perceived roles of men in society?

This is what we need to start showing teenage boys, as well as those who are trying to persuade them not to enter the nursing profession.

We let teenage boys decide whether they want to become nurses through **collaborative teaching.** You want to show these young men that there are other 'manly men' in the profession. Having some talks surrounding the nursing occupation delivered primarily by men is the perfect starting point. One needs to allow teenage boys to believe that their role as male nurses is coveted and respected and not a sign of femininity.

Another way to introduce teenage boys to the nursing profession is by allowing schools the opportunity to visit universities that have **simulation labs**. Let already qualified male nurses show them the exciting aspect of nursing - the procedures that you get to perform at the bedside. With that, give the teenage boys a taste of what they can expect and the different routes they can follow as male nurses.

Nursing doesn't have to be restricted to a patient's bedside. Male nurses can enlist in the military, obtain a qualification in emergency medicine, and even scrub in and play a pivotal role in the success of surgeries. You want teenage boys to see the degree of excitement that the prospect of male nursing will offer them.

At career fairs, make sure that there is a male nurse with a stand. Let them see that the profession exists. This in-person interaction and sharing of lived experiences with other qualified registered nurses will ensure that more teenage boys start to consider this rewarding profession.

In 2011, less than three percent of registered nurses were male. That said, as of 2021, that number has increased to 13.7%. Teenage boys need to be encouraged to move against the grain and follow where their passions lie. Not everyone needs to become a doctor, and, to be honest, any healthcare system would fail and crash without nurses. Their importance should, therefore, not be discounted.

There is also a specific stereotype that there are no jobs within the nursing field and that it is nearing saturation. This statement is untrue, and male nurses can still enjoy a stable career, professional growth opportunities, and a competitive salary.

In many societies, men are still seen as the primary breadwinners of the house. Becoming a male nurse will enable you to do that, as well as be able to save lives in the process. It is this level of satisfaction that a man yearns for, and teen boys need to be made aware of this.

The profession of nursing is more than changing bedpans and checking vitals. The various fields in nursing mean that boys will have a wide variety of choices depending on what they want to do. They can get to travel, for example, if they become field nurses, or work in the emergency room if they choose to become an ER nurse, and so on.

Aside from the traditional responsibilities, these different specialties also mean that there is a wide variety of challenges they will encounter and overcome, making it a very fulfilling career that could give one a sense of purpose.

Debunking the Stereotypes

It is crucial as a parent to teach your child that the stereotypes around male nurses perpetuated by TV shows should not keep them from pursuing nursing. The ideas on the TV shows about men in nursing are outdated, and boys should know just as much. But it is not enough to simply tell them that the ideas on these shows are inaccurate. Seek shows with positive representation of men in nursing as a replacement for the negative views. Provide the perfect ground for your son to take up an interest in nursing.

There has been a lot of concerted effort to get women into professions that men previously dominated. Therefore, there is no reason why men cannot get into a profession that was once thought of as only for women. Besides, the gender stereotypes and biases around nursing are a recent phenomenon, and men and nursing go way back, as we will see later in this book.

Let young boys understand that men and nursing are just as good a combination as women and nursing, and let them know the history of men in the profession. So, to put your sons into a position where they do not get negatively affected by the opposing views towards men in nursing, getting them to look at men positively in the profession is the best.

Practically Speaking

Work with male nurses in the family to offer a positive influence when they are still young. If there is a male relative who is a nurse, have them constantly speak to your son about the nursing profession. If you, as the father, are the nurse, be a positive influence on him. Show him the positive side of being a nurse. Answer any questions your son poses. As they grow, they might ask some more challenging questions; be honest in answering them too.

But ensure your child has the best possible positive impact from male nurses around them so that they have no doubts about wanting to get into the field when they grow up despite the setbacks.

Men are not born naturally bad at caring and nurturing. Instead, this trait is something that they learn as boys because that is what society teaches them men should be. Men can just be as caring, nurturing, and empathetic as women. They are just as kind and reliable.

Thus, introducing them to nursing at that tender age works well in making them grow up having internalized the fact that they are just as caring and nurturing as women. This makes it much easier for them to then join the nursing field than if they grow up with negative gender biases and have to fight them in adulthood.

Gender stereotypes are not started and perpetuated in a vacuum. They are imprinted on us in childhood, and even when we know better as adults, changing them is hard. Thus, start your sons early in gaining a positive view of nursing, and they will have no doubts about the profession as adults – the earlier, the better.

Chapter 2: High School and College Decisions

If you aren't entirely apt to understand how to get into nursing, there will be a few things that you will need to take into consideration. From your academic performance to the subjects you should consider taking in high school, we will outline the bare minimum and the different types of nursing programs on offer.

Your academic performance is of great importance in high school. The better you perform, the greater your chances of getting into your dream college. However, that also does not mean you must get 100% for all your tests and assignments. You will need to look at each of the nursing courses that are on offer at a variety of different colleges. Some colleges may require a Grade-Point Average (GPA) of more than 3.3, whereas others may only consider your application with a score higher than 3.5.

With academic performance comes a myriad of other factors, such as the extracurriculars you did at school and the subjects you specialized in. Usually applying for nursing will usually require science-based subjects such as chemistry, physics, and biology. For this reason, you want to ensure that you study at a high school that provides these subjects.

This is why students who want to become male nurses are always encouraged to do extracurricular activities over and above, devoting time and effort to their academics. In many cases, when applying to colleges, there are students with the same GPA who can only be differentiated based on the number of extracurricular activities they were a part of. If this is the same as well, the next step would be scrutinizing the college essays submitted along with your application.

When writing your college admission essay, if required, you need to showcase your strengths in a way that shows vulnerability, strength, and dedication to becoming a male nurse. You want the college admission boards to be unable to find a reason to reject your application.

With that being said, having multiple iterations of your essay that can adapt to different colleges is always a fantastic approach to take. The reason for various iterations is that you want to show the admissions board that you have researched their college and that it isn't just a run-of-the-mill decision.

Now, let's jump into the different nursing courses you will encounter when applying to colleges. Not all of the colleges offer all the varieties of nursing qualifications, which is why you want to make sure you are applying for the nursing route of your choice in an institute that offers the course.

Here are a few of the nursing courses that are present in the college database:

- **A Licensed Practical Nurse (LPN)** qualification is only one year long and acts as an excellent bridging course to becoming a Registered Nurse (RN). You can even use this course to dabble in the nursing field and see what it means to be a male nurse.

During this course, you will be supervised by an RN. This will provide the perfect platform for you to obtain insights from someone who has been a part of the profession for quite some time. Depending on which college you attend, most will require your SAT scores or TOEFL if you are an international student interested in studying to become a male nurse.

- **The Associate Degree in Nursing (ADN)** focuses more on the technical aspects of the nursing career, taking up to two years to complete. Offered throughout many colleges and community colleges, an ADN can treat and provide education to patients. This can be seen as the second step if you found the LPN rather intriguing!

- **A Bachelor of Science in Nursing (BSN)** is a four-year degree program offered at many colleges. With this qualification, you will delve into the clinical arena of being a nurse, focusing on the bedside management of patients, as well as being a part of a multidisciplinary healthcare team. Not only is this degree internationally recognized, but it provides a good starting salary. The former and latter are both critical to men, especially the breadwinners of their households.

With these three qualifications being the most common, some programs allow for extra coursework to be completed, allowing for a transition from an RN to a BSN. Most of the male nurses who choose this route enjoy the freedom it allows them to study and earn a salary at the same time. However, at this point, you may be asking, "Is this as far as I can go?" The quick and most correct answer is 'no.'

Once you've obtained your BSN, you can apply for a Master's in Nursing, allowing you to enter into a specialized nursing field, which can range from a Neonatal Nurse Practitioner (NNP) to a Pediatric Nurse Practitioner (PNP) or even a Nurse Educator (NE).

Do you like the field of anaesthesiology? Well, there is even a Certified Registered Nurse Anaesthetist (CRNA) qualification that can be done.

Also, you can pursue a Master's in Nursing, the Master's of Science in Nursing (MSN). This is a non-clinical graduate-level degree aimed at improving your leadership skills so that you are much more likely to be promoted. To pursue an MSN, you often need to be an RN with a BSN. With a Master's, you put yourself in a better position to then get into leadership positions.

Job opportunities you can get with an MSN include Chief Nursing Officer, Patient Care Director, Clinical Nurse Leader, and Nurse Practitioner. Other specialized roles will include Nurse Educator and Nurse Informatics Specialist. So, if you feel like you can and want to go further, then the MSN is the best route after completing your BSN.

Mentorship

One way to put yourself in an excellent position in the nursing profession is to consider mentorship. Since most men in nursing actually want more men to join them in the field, they are very open to mentorship programs for male high school students who wish to get into nursing.

These programs can be found all across various states and even in your local area. A quick google search can help you with this.

Such programs have several benefits, chief among which is that they provide support, guidance, and assistance to male nurses and nursing students. The nursing mentorships can help you create contacts, which will be critical in helping you find someone you can shadow to learn more about the profession.

Aside from that, mentorship also helps you understand the emotional labor of nursing and prepare for it. Nursing requires you to manage your emotions well while interacting with patients, colleagues and others in a professional setting. Thus, male nurses can help you learn how to navigate this reality before you even begin training.

Another situation is that, while male nurses are marginalized, the marginalization is worse for Black, Hispanic, and other marginalized communities' male students. According to statistics published in Minority Nurse.com, only 24.7 % of Registered nurses are from a minority group.

 The remaining percentage is filled by male nurses who identify as White. This 24.7% is not bad, but you must consider that several ethnicities and races exist. Only 9.9% are African American/Black; 8.3% are Asians; 4.8% are Latino or Hispanic; 1.3% consider themselves as two or more races, and 0.4% are American Indians.

So, besides dealing with gender stereotypes directed at men in nursing, male nurses from the marginalized and minorities also have to deal with racial and ethnic stereotypes. Many male nurses from these communities have shared their stories of navigating the workplace while also dealing with gender and racial stereotypes.

When such nurses find themselves in this position, they are double minorities, and this situation can make their work environment extremely difficult to navigate. Mental breakdown, job dissatisfaction, and depression can kick in and make these nurses either quit or stop giving their best in a job where they always need to give their best.

The situation worsens when you consider that several studies have found that minority nurses, men or women, are underpaid and often under-recognized.

Due to the issues mentioned above, it is crucial that male student nurses join mentorship programs that deal with the unique situation of being a nurse from a minority group.

For example, the National Black Nurse Association (NBNA) provides a professional voice for over 200,000 African American nurses across the U.S. The NBNA caters to both men and women, but it does have nursing mentorship programs catered exclusively to men.

Asian American and Pacific Islander (AAPI) provides mentorship for all nurses of Asian descent, including male nurses. For Hispanics, the National Association of Hispanic Nurses (NAHN) caters to nurses of Hispanic descent.

All these organizations provide mentorship programs that help male nursing students acquire knowledge and understanding of the nursing profession. They also create contact with experienced nurses who can take them under their wing and be their guiding light in the profession.

Other professional groups that can also help you get more comfortable in the profession are the American Nurses Association, National Student Nursing Association, Brotherhood of Nursing, and the American Association of Men in Nursing. By being proactive and joining these associations, you are making it much easier for yourself to settle into the profession. Social integration and sharing knowledge and skills mean that you set yourself up for success in the field.

As you can see, the decisions you make in high school may directly impact the route you take when deciding to become a male nurse.

However, once you have your foot in the door, you will have a wealth of opportunities at your fingertips!

Chapter 3: Best Fields in Nursing for Men

While we look at nursing as a single profession, it is a very broad field with many sub-categories to select from, depending on your interests, strengths, skills, and prospects.

The fields below are mentioned because they have a high ratio of men, which can make your integration into the nursing profession a lot easier. At the end of the day, however, the best field is the one you feel most passionate about.

1. Emergency Room Nurse

Becoming an emergency room nurse will put you in a fast-paced, ever-changing environment, but it is one of the best-paying nursing jobs you can find. About 19.8% of ER nurses are male, which is higher than the average.

To become an ER nurse, you will need an associate's degree in nursing (ASN) or a Bachelor of Science in Nursing (BSN). You then will become licensed by passing the National Councils Licensure Examination for registered nurses (NCLEX-RN).

An ER nurse's primary responsibilities include taking a patient's vital signs, administering medicine prescribed by the doctor, helping provide treatment, and monitoring the patient as they recover.

2. Intensive Care Unit (ICU) Nurse

The ICU field has 18.2 percent of men. To become an ICU nurse, you will need to complete your AND or BSN and pass your NCLEX-RN exam.

There are further sub-categories that you can specialize in as an ICU nurse, including:

- Neonatal ICU nurse (working with newborn babies faced with life-threatening conditions)

- Neuroscience ICU nurse (caring for patients who have had a stroke due to a blood clot in the brain)

- Surgical/trauma ICU nurse (caring for patients who are unstable or ill and in need of surgery. You will also care for such patients once they are out of the theatre)

- Medical ICU (caring for patients with critical illness but do not require surgery, such as patients with Respiratory Distress Syndrome, Diabetic patients, patients suffering from liver cirrhosis, etc.)

3. Nurse anesthetist

Sometimes referred to as a Certified Registered Nurse Anesthetist (CRNA), about 41 percent of nurse anesthetists are men, so you are guaranteed to have many male colleagues in this field. This field also takes the most time, with 6-8 years spent in higher education.

Your primary responsibilities will be to prepare patients and then administer anesthesia, maintain the anesthesia through the operation, and then as the patient recovers. Your work schedule and demands while on the job will vary depending on where you work. If you work in an environment with a high number of surgeries, you will be quite busy.

Nurse anesthetists are one of the most in-demand nurses in healthcare. Thus, if you train and specialize in this, you set yourself up for tons of job openings. Due to the extended education period, it is also the highest-paying nursing field, as you expect an average salary of $195,610 or more.

4. Flight nurse

If you wish to work in nursing but also experience the thrill of traveling while on the job, then becoming a flight nurse is a field you should consider. Male flight nurses are about 18%.

As a flight nurse, you will deliver critical care to patients while traveling in an aircraft to the hospital or any other setting.

No matter how thrilling it sounds, this job will still demand a lot from you. First, providing airborne care is challenging; thus, experience is crucial if you want to succeed in the field. At least five years' experience in a similar setting is needed to become a flight nurse.

You should also be able to handle high-pressure situations as you will most often be dealing with patients facing life-or-death circumstances.

5. Rehabilitation nurse

You require an Associate's Degree in Nursing or a Bachelor of Science in Nursing to be a rehabilitation nurse. Working as a rehabilitation nurse means that you specialize in helping people recovering from serious illnesses or people with disabilities attain proper function or health of their body or help them adapt to a new altered lifestyle. About 28 percent of rehabilitation nurses are men, so you will be in great company.

As a rehabilitation nurse, you will not be limited to hospitals. You can work in long-term healthcare facilities, inpatient and outpatient rehabilitation centers, schools, private practice, and community and home healthcare environments. This means then that you choose the best place where you can enjoy your profession.

As a rehab nurse, you will not only work with the patients but also with their families and caregivers at the onset of a disability or injury. This means you will need to display very high emotional intelligence, have excellent interpersonal skills, and be calm and patient.

6. Nurse practitioner

Working as a nurse practitioner means that you are conferred more authority than a registered nurse and will even be assigned similar responsibilities to those of a doctor. To qualify for this post, however, you need to complete a Master's of Science in Nursing or a Doctor of Nursing Practice.

Only 13.1% of nurse practitioners are men, so entering into this field means that you will be adding to the number of men in the field, as there is a real demand for more men to take up positions in this sector.

As a nurse practitioner, your main responsibilities will be managing overall patient care, diagnosing and even treating chronic and acute illnesses such as diabetes, HBP, infections, and injuries, educating patients and families on disease prevention, and guiding them on positive health and lifestyle choices.

Good interpersonal communication, emotional intelligence, and empathy are the core of the family nurse practitioner because your average day will mostly be spent meeting and examining patients, answering questions, and making consultations with physicians. You might also have plenty of paperwork, but you will spend a lot more time with patients.

You can also become a psychiatric nurse practitioner, which means you specialize in mental health and, thus, work with patients that suffer from psychiatric disorders.

The nurse practitioner field is among the highest-paying nursing fields, with the U.S Bureau of Labor Statistics putting the medium pay at $ 123,780 as of 2021.

7. Public health nurse

Public health nurses are the largest professional segment of the healthcare profession, let alone the nursing profession.

This cadre of nurses plays a critical role in improving the health outcomes of a give population because their primary responsibilities involve educating the community on health care, including prevention of common diseases, advocacy, activism, and evaluation of public health.

In health facilities, a public health nurse is responsible for recording and analyzing medical data, evaluating patients, creating treatment plans, and working with physicians to deliver top-quality care.

To work as a public health nurse, you need to complete your course to become a registered nurse. After this, you can then choose to become a public health nurse based on your desire to effect direct change in your community.

The above fields are some of the best ones you can consider when entering nursing. But remember to follow what you want, even if it is not a male-dominated field. Your presence in a nursing field very few men are in could be the spark it needs to get more men into it. Be a trailblazer, and do not be shy about it. Be proud that you are doing something that will be considered to have opened the path for many other men that came after you.

Chapter 4: Scholarship Programs for Male Nurses

Some scholarship programs target men in nursing and help you go through your nursing education smoothly. These programs make it easier for men to study any field in nursing, acting as a bridge between male nursing students and the profession. They include:

1. The American Association of Men in Nursing

This body offers mentorship to nurses and male student nurses and also provides scholarships across the country for men looking to enter the field. The association aims to provide men with resources to help them enter the profession so that it meets its goal of enhancing male presence in the field.

Their annual AAMN scholarship is open to all male students enrolled in a nursing program and are seeking scholarship opportunities. The AAMN considers your application and your academic standings.

2. Hector Gonzalez Past Presidents Scholarship

Hector Gonzalez Past Presidents Scholarship is offered by the National Association of Hispanic Nurses and caters to Hispanic male nurses. The scholarship program aims to encourage the men of the Hispanic population to continue and complete their nursing program to increase the ethnic group's presence in the field.

Another scholarship targeted towards Hispanics is the **Hispanic Scholarship Fund**, which looks at your GPA scores, among other criteria.

3. Men in Nursing Scholarship

The Men in Nursing Award provides the Men in Nursing Scholarship, which The Great Nurse Foundation supplies. The scholarship is given twice a year.

However, to qualify for this scholarship, you need to be a member and also be enrolled in an accredited nursing program. When writing your application, you must include a written submission regarding the male nurses' situation and the barriers you face in the industry.

4. Scholarships for black male nurses

The National Black Nurses Association also provides scholarships for black male nurses. The organization has thirteen scholarship opportunities, with each program having its own specific criteria. They are also dispersed to the students based on the applicant's academic merit, their current standings in their programs, and future goals in their nursing career. Some of these programs will also require you to be enrolled in specific programs to qualify, for example, graduate or undergraduate programs.

5. NurseTim

NurseTim is a scholarship program aimed at male nurses who are in a nursing program at any level. Aside from academic performance, the level of service the applicant offers is also considered. Thus, to qualify, you not only need to be good in class but also be active in the field.

6. Breaking Barriers

Breaking Barriers Scholarship for Men in Nursing is targeted to male nurses and students who may be U.S residents but also have a legal permanent residency and majoring in nursing. You must also hold a 3.5 GPA score and write a 500-1000 word-essay.

7. Emergency Nurse Association

Emergency Nurse Association (ENA) Foundation Academic Scholarship is explicitly aimed at nurses specializing in emergency care, helping them with a scholarship opportunity in their career program.

These scholarships are in a variety, including some which are open to men who live outside the U.S and desire to become emergency nurses. Members of ENA will often be open to applying to all levels of scholarships, while nonmembers will only be allowed to apply for undergraduate funding.

8. HRSA Nurse Corps

This society is unique in that the amount you get in your scholarship will depend on whether you agree to work in areas with critical needs of nurses. This means that to qualify for the scholarship, you need to be in a situation where you can move to your work facility upon graduation. Thus, you need to have no existing service commitment.

The scholarship covers education costs – tuition, books, and lab fees. Still, they also provide financial assistance to recipients enrolled in an accredited and recognized nursing program within the U.S.

9. Army Nurse Corps

Army Nurse Corps Association Scholarship is for military men in the nursing program. It is targeted at men who are enrolled in a Bachelor's or advanced nursing degree and could either be active or a veteran.

Among the requirements to apply is that retired veterans need to have been Honorably Discharged from the military.

10. AAPINA

The Asian American/Pacific Islander Nurses Association (AAPINA) Scholarship is aimed at Asian Americans, and Pacific Islanders pursuing an undergrad or graduate nursing degree.

The scholarship is open to members who have been with the organization for two years and have a 3.5 and above GPA academic score. An applicant will also need to write an essay on their leadership potential.

The above scholarships are a great way for you to take the initiative and be the master of your own destiny. Not only will these scholarships help you complete your nursing program, but some can help you further your education in your chosen sector, meaning an increased potential to earn more.

Chapter 5: Parent Myths About Male Nursing

We cannot underestimate our parents' influence on our future careers. Some individuals first need approval from their parents before sending in their college applications. This makes it very difficult for high school students to apply for majors and degrees that go against the grain.

One of those that do go against the grain is male nursing. This is primarily due to the myths that surround male nursing.

Here we are going to be discussing a few of them, as well as debunking them in the process.

1. It's a women's profession

The one central myth is that nursing is purely a woman's profession. Although the number of male nurses is increasing, it must be understood that both male and female nurses can coexist within the profession.

A fun fact is that your so-called 'manly men,' the burly policemen and firemen, will most likely migrate into the nursing field as a second career after retiring. If you think of it, it makes sense! Being a policeman or fireman means you are going to be a form of caretaker for the public, which fits very well within the notion of being a male nurse.

The job in itself is also rewarding for men, over and above the flexibility that can exist within the schedule and the excellent pay one receives.

2. The emotions factor

Another common myth that male nurses need to deal with is that men are seen as not emotionally suited to be a nurse. Now parents may also feel that a man's emotions cannot care for patients to the extent that female nurses do.

However, caring for others, being selfless, and being able to assist them with their physical functions are all related to being human, not necessarily a man. Yes, men may have more muscles to help with lifting patients and helping with broken bones in the emergency center, but they also have the clinical and mental aptitude for devising a care plan at the same level as any female nurse.

3. The other option

Nursing is seen as a 'catch-22,' that is, as a field where those rejected from medical school migrate. This is an entirely incorrect perception!

Any healthcare system would collapse without the presence of nurses. That is just a fact, with there being no research that can prove otherwise. This is how parents need to think about their sons when they express their desire to become male nurses.

Parents want their children to be change agents, and being a male nurse provides you with the strength to prevent a pivotal system from entirely collapsing on itself.

4. Stereotypical

Another contentious myth that needs to be debunked is that all male nurses are homosexuals. We live in a day and age where our parents still maintain these stereotypes, especially when gender fluidity has been explained en masse.

Men are stereotypically seen as being strong and firm, whereas the perception of the nursing field is that you are gentle, show emotion, and care for others. The latter, believe it or not, exists within a male nurse's repertoire without them needing to be labeled as a homosexual. Remember, just because a man is considered strong and firm does not necessarily mean they will always take on tough jobs. Thought-provoking, isn't it?

That said, nursing is still a job that requires physical and mental stamina, so the thought that when a man takes up nursing, they are taking up a soft job is a myth. The view that nursing is soft is rooted in the fact that it has mostly been a field for women; since women are viewed as soft.

While the different specialty fields in nursing will need different levels of physical stamina and mental fortitute, the reality is that all nursing fields will require physical and mental stamina at varying levels.

There are long working hours, working with people with nasty injuries and wounds, and constantly being alert to patients under your care. Additionally, the male nurses will be the ones called to do the heavy lifting of patients or hospital equipment. So, nursing is, indeed, a tough job for male nurses.

Furthermore, nurses are the first line of contact between patients and doctors. Being the first line of contact means you are at a greater risk of contracting infectious diseases if the patients are suffering from them.

With the COVID-19 pandemic still lingering, various studies are coming out revealing that nurses are the healthcare workers who got the most infections of the illness (at over 50% infections). It takes great strength and courage to put yourself in the line of danger to take care of and keep other people alive.

Indeed, if you as a parent are worried about your son getting into a field that will be too soft for them, nursing is not one of them. In fact, be proud that your son is taking on a job that puts them directly in the line of fire because it is a sign of their strength and bravery.

5. Is anyone hiring?

As a parent, you want to ensure that your son enters a profession where job opportunities will always be available. Some parents believe that male nurses won't get hired as much as female nurses. In actuality, many facilities prefer male nurses based on their strength and physique! They lift patients more efficiently and can assist them in the bathroom or when they need to be turned in their beds.

Nursing is an exhausting profession, and it is promised that male nurses will work just as hard, if not harder, than their female counterparts. Naturally, men are also statistically better suited to handle trauma and critical cases!

It is challenging to interact with parents who believe myths more than they do the potential and passions their children have. However, constantly contesting their perceived notions of their young men wanting to become male nurses provides an intrinsic cognitive shift that they will be able to use to change the thought processes of others (especially parents) who may think and feel the same way about their sons.

It is also improbable for male nurses to be insignificant in the nursing profession, even with prevailing gender stereotypes. There is nothing about being a man in a field dominated by women that is insignificant. So, even if a male nurse wanted to be insignificant, the prevailing cultural outlook towards male nurses means they will stand out even in situations they do not want to.

So, perhaps as a parent, your concern should be whether your son can handle the constant scrutiny that comes with being a male nurse rather than them being insignificant. The truth is, men in nursing are usually under a lot of scrutiny, and the confidence of still going about their job despite this is what makes successful male nurses.

So you see, parents, being a male nurse doesn't mean that your son will be treated insignificantly or that they will be worse off in terms of their future in the nursing field. In actual fact, there may even be a few more opportunities that they would benefit more from than female nurses.

So, give your sons the benefit of the doubt and support them in their career-making decisions. Trust us; the support will go further than them being unhappy in a profession they have no passion for.

Chapter 6: The Sad Truth Most Male Nurses Fear

There is this predisposed notion that having a healing touch comes from a woman. Using this thought with feminine imagery to describe the nursing profession has allowed it to be seen as a field just for women.

A fun fact is that most nurses were actually males in ancient times. It was only as we entered the 19th century that there was a marked shift in the gender composition of nurses. But, what remains a sad truth is that men still fear *if they should become nurses in today's day and age.*

Primarily, the stigma of being a part of the profession may classify a male nurse as more feminine. Not to mention the degree of ambiguity regarding their social status and the disapproval that may come from their friends and family. Because of this, 85% of dropouts from the nursing profession are men. This is in comparison to the 35% that are women. Some people will even go as far as to say those male nurses are your typical misfits and were unable to secure a place in any other profession.

The myths of men being bad at nursing may well have been believed long before her, but Florence Nightingale probably had the most significant influence in pushing men from nursing. While she knew of and even interacted with male nurses, when she established her nursing school at the St Thomas Hospital in

London, she only welcomed women into her three-year education in nursing.

Men who were accepted were only taken in due to their physical strengths. And even then, they would often get a lower level of education than the women and would then be tasked with caring only for the mentally ill patients in psychiatric hospitals. They were never let into general hospital care.

Times are Tough

Just think of how taboo it may seem if male nurses were to be hired for the delivery room. The notions that many females hold against men regarding their possible experience of women objectification have entirely eliminated the chances of some men heading into specific specialties.

Contrastingly, male nurses are expected to be able to function in high-stress environments such as the Emergency Department (ED) or Intensive Care Unit (ICU).

These stereotypes against male nurses are perpetuated by the media on a daily basis. For example, the movie 'Meet the Parents,' featuring Ben Stiller, depicts him as a nurse and the intense ridicule that followed his choice of profession. To be honest, these thoughts about male nurses ostracize them, causing many to feel the need to defend their masculinity, completely withdrawing themselves from interacting with their female coworkers.

There is also the 'touch' aspect of the nursing profession, which may not be as easy for male nurses to execute. In many cases, men are stereotyped and stigmatized based on being sexual aggressors and more capable of committing sexual misconduct.

This means that even the most respectful touch to merely comfort a patient might be seen as physical harassment by a patient should it be a male nurse, compared to a female counterpart. A pitfall in the nursing education system is that male nurses aren't necessarily equipped to tackle this gender conflict, as they are trained from a less transformative aspect that tends more toward the female perspective.

The myth of the "touch" also grew in popularity during the late 1800s. Since men were only allowed a lower level of nursing education, many could not get into general hospital practice. In fact, men in Nightingale's nursing school who wanted to expand their learning into general hospital practice, and especially into maternal-child nursing, were often viewed as perverts and would even be expelled if they persisted. This perception took hold and is still perpetuated even today, hence why the touch of male nurses is still viewed with suspicion.

What about female nurses?

However, although we are aware of the stigma that males experience, what about female nurses accepting males into what is deemed to be their profession? Female nurses may expect more traditional tasks, such as intense physical lifting, to be undertaken by male nurses.

However, female nurses may feel that male nurses are trying to establish a stronghold within their profession, resulting in a possible backlash against male nurses entering the profession.

With many unknowns due to the lack of male nurses currently in the field, only time will tell. However, should issues arise that establish a gender power struggle, there will always be a solution.

To help encourage men to enter the nursing profession, it is vital to tackle the stereotypical media portrayals that exist regarding male nurses. High school guidance counselors can start at the base of the problem by debunking these myths when interacting with students interested in the field. This is one of the only ways we can create an environment encouraging male nurses to work with female nurses at the patient's bedside.

It's an inside job

There need to be more concerted efforts from male nurses towards debunking the negative perceptions around them in the field. Men simply being in the field is not enough.

In fact, it is just the start of the long journey toward changing the perception of male nurses in nursing. Male nurses need to go out of their way to ensure that everyone they interact with or come into contact with has something positive to say about them.

It is hard to change the view that men are rough and not built for the nursing field. Still, by constantly being a positive influence on everyone you come across, by continually showing people your vulnerable and emotional side, your fears of getting judged or viewed simply through your gender lenses diminish.

People soon become aware that you are simply a nurse doing anything that a nurse can and should do, regardless of gender. Do not let the fear of stigmatization or ridicule stop you from doing anything you want in nursing. You are a man who is simply doing his job in a field that you chose; your gender is beyond you.

Male nurses bring a completely different perspective to the operations of nursing. With their different approach to the field, it can only result in a strengthening of the core values that nurses hold within the medical fraternity. Although the presence of male nurses is on the rise, it is believed that both the patients and the rest of the multidisciplinary healthcare team will benefit from an increased gender balance.

Chapter 7: Male Nursing Requires a Confident and Positive Choice

So you have decided to become a male nurse? This is such a fantastic decision! Although we are in your corner cheering you on, we need to emphasize that you need to be 120% confident in your choice. As a male nurse, you may have already experienced some form of resistance from others regarding your choice. Unfortunately, the patients and coworkers you'll be working with may share the same views.

This is why it is essential to be confident in your decision to become a male nurse and ensure that purely positive intentions drive your passion. As we delve into our confidence, we can feel ready for the experiences that life is about to show us. This is important for male nurses because not only will you be learning a completely new field, but you will be shaping the field by just being present in the class.

There will be opportunities for immense growth in the nursing profession. By ensuring you have enough confidence to tackle and grasp these opportunities, you are providing yourself with a degree of personal and professional growth.

The reality is that you will have periods of self-doubt during your studies, not because you are a male but because it is a normal process of attending college. It sounds horrible, but it is the unfortunate reality of being a college student. Confidence in your decision to become a male nurse ensures that you are ready to face these challenges head-on and rise above them.

When you enter any part of the healthcare field, you need to make sure you have a positive mindset about the profession. You need to have that passion that nobody can quell, no matter how hard they try.

Yes, being a male nurse will come with quite a stable salary and even the opportunity to specialize as a travel nurse, pediatric nurse, or a nurse primed for the emergency department. But, you cannot thrive in the profession by looking purely at the materialistic benefits of the profession. The nursing fraternity is at a point where they need passionate male nurses who want to change the face of the nursing profession for the better.

Indeed, a view of only material benefits could be a hindrance to getting into the field because it could be a sign that someone overlooks or underplays the challenges they will encounter when they enter nursing. While male nurses earn significantly a lot more, the reality is that the challenges they encounter at work make them more likely to negotiate for higher pay.

So, sure, you want to get into nursing because you will get a good salary, but are you ready to put in extra shifts?

Are you ready to work for long hours, sometimes even a whole 24 hours?

Are you ready to do a lot of heavy lifting when called upon, which will be a lot of times?

Are you ready to take the ridicule that comes with being male in a female-dominated field and still maintain your focus?

Are you ready to face a work environment where you might become socially isolated?

The above questions might make it seem like they are intended to intimidate you, but nothing could be further from the truth. Being honest with yourself about the work environment you will encounter will shape your attitude when entering that field. Simply believing that becoming a male nurse will be easy since the pay is good is not the attitude that will help you settle in your job. If anything, when pay becomes your primary objective in becoming a male nurse, you probably won't last long in the profession to enjoy the full benefits of that good paycheck.

By entering nursing as a man, you are choosing to go into a field that, while not hostile to men, is still deeply rooted in gender biases and stereotypes. You will constantly be reminded of your gender; you will encounter snarky comments about your masculinity, and you could be taken off some responsibilities simply because you are a man.

Are you ready to face all that? If yes, your confidence and positive attitude will shape you for future success.

Nonetheless, by becoming a male nurse, you will be a beacon of hope for many other male high schoolers who want to take the leap into the nursing profession. You need to be able to trust in yourself and that you are going to make a difference. Once you believe that you can do that and inspire the next generation of male nurses, you will understand why this profession is the best fit for you.

But what if you struggle with being confident, especially when challenged by family and friends regarding your decision? Well, you need to start by creating a confident mindset. This is where you shake off self-doubt and retrain your brain to convert any "I can't" to "I can." When you combine this with remembering your 'why,' you will be destined for success as a male nurse.

But remember to always be yourself! Given the high-stress healthcare environment, allowing the profession to change you is problematic. Dare to be the real you! As a male nurse, cry when you need to cry, rejoice when you get to perform your first procedures, and don't allow others' perceptions of your choices to define your destiny.

Chapter 8: Role Models in Nursing

Role models in nursing go as far back as when males were the predominant gender within the profession. And as current male high schoolers may face scrutiny with choosing to become a male nurse, the same degree of scrutiny was experienced by these historical male nurses.

They were all regarded as incapable of establishing a proper patient relationship. Still, they rose above and beyond these assumptions, overcoming copious amounts of rejection and unfair treatment to become the role models that they are today.

1. Camillus de Lellis

Camillus de Lellis is the first male nurse role model that we will look at. Now, he may be well-renowned as a patron saint for nurses worldwide, but he is also the first-ever male nurse to enter the profession. He overcame gambling, aggression, and rejection and became the hospital director in a hospital that had once denied his application to become the first-ever male nurse.

He was more than just a man who had done his mandatory military service. He cared for both the dying and the sick with a degree of empathy that was unmatched by many female nurses. During his gambling escapades, he dabbled in a bit too much alcohol. He used his own recovery as a template to help others who were also fighting alcoholism.

St. Camillus found himself on the battlefield, helping to mend those who were forced into wars they never wanted to be a part of. He reassured the ill, developed the first ambulance service, and created a hospital that was primarily directed at assisting alcoholics. St. Camillus was known to be able to think out of the box, much like male nurses are required to do today!

Also, did you know that St. Camillus inspired the symbol of the Red Cross, which we still use today? During his service to humanity in Rome, St. Camillus founded the male monastic order of the Camillians, a group of male nurses who cared for the sick and dying. The Camillians used the symbol of the Red Cross to identify them as the order of male caregivers. This symbol is what we use today to refer to healthcare.

As we see, men's influence in healthcare, especially nursing, is not to be taken for granted.

2. Edward T. Lyon

It was in 1955 that the second most well-renowned role model would make an appearance. His name was 2nd Lieutenant Edward T. Lyon. Now, although he was not the first male nurse known to man, he was the first male nurse to be enlisted into the Army Nurse Corps in the United States.

He was an anesthetist nurse right before joining the Corps, along with more than 3,500 female nurses. It was how he excelled that motivated many other men to become male nurses in the military corps.

However, although stereotypes had restricted male nurses from climbing the corporate ladder within the nursing field, Lyon definitely took the first step in making male nurse promotions possible!

3. Joe Hogan

With the number of males now being inspired to venture on the path of becoming male nurses, it was Joe Hogan who really made a mark. In the 1970s, he was one of the first African-American male nurses to fight for equal rights for those with a bachelor's degree in nursing.

Hogan found that he was starting to become discriminated against as a male, primarily because most universities were not accepting male students for the nursing program. It was in 1982 that his court case gained international traction, resulting in the abolishment of any gender-based discrimination clauses that some universities laid claim to.

Joe Hogan's win was also significant because he is a great role model to male nurses from marginalized communities who, aside from facing discrimination in nursing due to their gender, also face further discrimination due to their ethnicity or race.

Thus, his influence and presence provide men from marginalized communities hope that they will get to pursue a career they love and study it to the best of their ability.

4. Luther Christman

Luther Christman is a note role model who continuously fought to end discrimination against male nurses. He was denied acceptance into two different nursing programs because he was a man. He couldn't apply for maternal-specific nursing programs, with his rejections being based on nothing other than the fact that he is a male.

Christman wasn't going to allow this level of discrimination to harbor the future that he saw for himself, so he established the National Male Nursing Association, which was later renamed the American Assembly For Men in Nursing.

Christman was a man who advocated for male nurses to take up their rightful positions within the nursing field. He was able to encourage so many young men to venture into nursing as he became the first male nurse inducted as a dean of a nursing school in the United States.

5. Russell Tranbarger

While male nurses such as Lyon and Christman were very vocal about their unhappiness, especially when discriminated against, some preferred a quieter approach to combating injustice.

Russell Tranbarger was such a man, mentoring other male nurses and pruning them to success rather than making big, bold moves/statements on national radio stations. He used all of his teachings to co-author the book *Men in Nursing: History,*

Opportunities, and Challenges.

The success of this book and his selfless nature to all of his fellow male nurses resulted in him being inducted into the 2012 Hall of Fame for the American Nurses Association.

6. James Derham

James Derham, another role model, was born as a slave and worked as a male nurse whilst still being 'owned.' It was only after he was released from slavery that he went on to use his experience as a male nurse to become a physician!

His influence is even more significant among the African-American community and other marginalized groups because he was considered the first black nurse. Derham apprenticed under influential American Physician John Kearsley Mitchell. Kearsley Mitchell taught Derham everything he needed to know about compound medicine (medicine that involved mixing different compounds and ingredients), bedside mannerisms, and the basics of treating patients, especially throat care.

After being transferred twice, Derham received his freedom in New Orleans, where he opened up his own nursing practice. This is considered the first documented medical practice owned and run by a Black man.

7. LeRoy Craig

Another influential male nurse is LeRoy Craig. Craig spent most of his career not only in nursing but also as an activist and educator who sought to increase the recognition and opportunities for male nurses. Craig was instrumental in male nurses gaining access to the American Nurse Association. Up into 1940, the ANA had been adamant about admitting men into the association.

He also fought for and succeeded in getting the U.S government to recognize the professional status of male nurses. LeRoy Graig was firm in his belief that men could serve in many capacities and areas in nursing and was unrelenting in encouraging men to join nursing. He motivated his male nursing students to specialize in various nursing positions such as Institutional nursing, Industrial nursing, Private duty nursing, special field, and federal government services.

Craig went on to found the Pennsylvania Hospital School of Nursing for Men in 1914 and was its superintendent, becoming the first male to hold that position in the U.S. Through its 51-year history, the school of nursing graduated more than 550 male nurses before it was dissolved in 1965.

These men are trailblazers in the nursing profession and are people that we can look up to now. But remember that you are in such a position right now as a male nurse. While you might not have the influence or sway that some of the nurses mentioned here have, in your own way, you can become a role model for children in modern times.

There is a significant focus on finding role models in the nursing profession, but you should also understand that you need to be the role model. As men only make up 7% of the nursing profession in the United States, you will not meet too many men to look up to or work with. So, it is then crucial that you take the initiative and become the role model you would have liked to have.

Remember, even as a minority in the nursing profession, the spotlight is on you due to your gender. The perceptions around nursing and gender mean that you will not easily escape standing out, at least in the current times. Therefore, ensure that you conduct yourself in a way that boys interested in nursing or younger male nurse students can look up to. And when they come into the facility, be the one to take them under your wing and guide them through the workplace.

Potential and current male nurses must be reminded of what history and role models have to say about their profession. As you can see, many of these role models took completely different routes and made vast advancements in the male nursing domain. Whether it be fighting discrimination or understanding how to bring male nurses into the profession in the future, each one used their passion for changing how the world sees them!

You have the potential to do that and so much more; all you need to do is remain humble, empathetic, and passionate about your journey of being a male nurse.

Chapter 9: Why Patients Love a Male Nurse

Patients can be somewhat finicky individuals. I mean, after all, can we blame them? They are in a very vulnerable position and in many cases, need the assistance of nurses for the treatment plan to be successful. Now the typical aspects of a female nurse, such as being caring, loving, empathetic, and patient, are well identified from the patient perspective. However, why do patients really love a male nurse?

Well, let's take it from both the female and male perspectives.

The Female Perspective

So, let's say the patient is a female, and the nurse is a male. Now there may be the apparent female patients who want to make small talk with a male nurse because of their looks or fantastic bedside manners, but many female patients prefer male nurses because of their kindness.

Yes, this sounds very similar to a female nurse, so what is the difference in the type of kindness provided? Female patients say that male nurses listen more intently and often interrupt less than female nurses.

Sure, female patients may feel a bit embarrassed when it is bath time or when they need to be rolled over on the bed. Still, they say that male nurses are a lot more careful with their movements, check in more with how the patient is feeling, and make them feel as comfortable as possible.

Contrastingly, female patients have said that female nurses many a time do not show the same level of care and are a lot more vigorous in terms of bath rituals, many times raising their voices to a patient when they are immensely frustrated.

We have never heard of a male nurse raising their voice to a male or female patient. See, male nurses are a lot more down-to-earth than any societal speculations that people have, both within and outside the nursing profession.

Now, let's examine why male patients prefer interactions with male nurses.

The Male Perspective

For one, there is just a specific level of understanding and bonding that happens between males, which isn't as markedly present between females. But that's way too psychological for the confines of this book!

You see, male patients prefer male nurses because of mutual respect for modesty. Male patients may feel insecure about their bodies, and it's just that they don't feel comfortable being bathed or having their clothes changed by a female.

Male patients also find that they can relate better to male nurses than nurses of the opposite sex. There are just some things a man can say to a man but not to a woman. Now it isn't because male patients don't trust the abilities of a female nurse; it's just difficult to explain some issues (e.g., erectile dysfunction) to them without feeling awkward. Men are just more comfortable with a more masculine approach to caring, such as playful teasing, rather than the more maternal approach female nurses use.

Young boys will also often be more open and confident speaking to male nurses because they relate to them more than they would with female nurses. Remember, as they grow into adolescence, young boys will often become somewhat shy of the opposite gender.

So, in a medical situation, they might find it harder to explain exactly what is wrong with their body to a female nurse, even when whatever is going on is not precisely embarrassing. Thus, they prefer to speak to a male nurse and will happily reveal the medical condition they are dealing with to them, making diagnosis and treatment easier.

Now, this next reason may sound rather far-fetched, but it is actually very true. Some religions may clash with a man's ability to be attended to by a female nurse. For example, men who practice Islam will require a male nurse to assist them during their hospital stay. You see, should there be a female nurse that oversees a male patient, and they are not seen as being related by either marriage or blood, it is a sin for them to be in the same enclosed space together. So this is another reason why male patients would prefer to have a male nurse assist them than a female nurse.

Sometimes, patients could simply love male nurses because they simply exceed expectations. Considering that many in society view men as less empathetic, less kind, and less caring when dealing with patients, they will often be blown away by their tenderness, kindness, and empathy. Perhaps, when patients who believe that men are less caring encounter male nurses who care and treat them with empathy, they are positively taken aback by this.

Thus, they might then view the male nurses as being more empathetic than female nurses. For such patients, they might ask for male nurses more since the men are challenging something that has been a core part of their belief for so long.

Another reason why patients love male nurses more is that male nurses will often be willing to share jokes and engage in banter from time to time with the patient. This is one of the ways male nurses display that they care. So, that sense of humor could also explain why patients would prefer a male nurse to care for them, as it makes them feel better too. This is not to say that female nurses are serious and don't engage in jokes. Rather, that male nurses will often be more inclined to use banter and jokes as their way of displaying their care.

There are so many more reasons why patients love to be treated by male nurses. They are committed to seeing their patients' progress, remain emotionally sound, and are less likely to allow their personal lives to impact how they act professionally.

Ultimately, a male nurse is a valued addition to any healthcare team, and stereotyping them based on preconceived notions hinders the nursing profession from evolving to the potential it is capable of.

Chapter 10: The Role of a Male Nurse Is Different Than One Would Think

Many aspects of being a male nurse may be seen as more tailored towards males than females. One of the key points related to this is the ability to advocate for the patients they will be treating. Male nurses have a more direct role of being able to advocate for patients who are unable to do so themselves. These could be children and those patients who do not have a parent or guardian. As mentioned before, male nurses are more inclined to **provide a listening ear.** Sometimes, all a patient wants is for you to listen, and this role is better suited to a male nurse.

The role of a male nurse can also be to provide that **male perspective** where necessary. For example, when male patients need to decide whether to get a vasectomy or not, a male nurse's perspective, when asked for it, may provide a bit more clarity on their decision.

Yes, a male nurse has a similar role to a female nurse's in creating a sound and safe place for patients to heal. This includes their **clinical tasks** such as taking vitals, performing diagnostic testing such as urine dipsticks and patient iron levels, and, depending on a nurse's specialty, emergency medicine or pediatric-specific tasks.

As a male nurse, you are **a role model for all young men** who want to move into the nursing field. You are their hope! You are also showing the world that men can also be nurturing and caring without needing to be classified as feminine!

A male nurse within the nursing space has a primary role of not only being an advocate for their patients but for males in general. Not only are there continuous streams of male-specific knowledge that are provided to them, but men's health issues become more relatable to the male nurse. Some female nurses may find this male-specific information useless because they are female, but this is where the problem arises. When female nurses do not take adequate care in understanding the male perspective, their male patients become disadvantaged.

The role of the male nurse is also to provide a **diversified healthcare environment.** Through increasing representation, and in this case, gender representation, you are allowing those 'macho men' who would otherwise be embarrassed to seek treatment due to female nurses to take their health into their own hands. Having male nurses within the profession encourages all types of patients to seek medical care.

We, unfortunately, live in a world where personal egos and stereotypes can act as a barrier to seeking healthcare and allowing your condition to worsen at home. Luckily for us, male nurses are rising and taking their place within the profession, breaking all these barriers and stereotypes one at a time!

Diversification of healthcare needs more men so that the unique way of caring that men display can be accommodated. We talked about the healing touch. Now, this is not to belabor the point of men's touch being considered perverse. Instead, the reality is that male nurses have learned to care for their patients differently.

If you look at how men act and interact with each other and the people they care for, they will often communicate their care through humor. So, male nurses will provide a much-needed light-hearted environment for patients, an environment of laughter and jokes, which is their way of displaying that they care.

This new outlook towards care is why we need more male nurses in the field because they open our eyes to new ways of caring for patients beyond simply giving them the healing touch. As the saying *'laughter is the best medicine'* implies, a male nurse will use their sense of humor to make a patient feel better as a female nurse uses her touch.

Male nurses can also be good **role models for young girls!** Yes, young girls can also look up to male nurses. Remember, when we talk of the stigmatization of male nurses at the workplace, young girls, just like young boys, are exposed to these during their childhood.

By providing positive views of male nurses to girls, you are also raising a generation of women who will see nothing strange with a man working as a nurse or even working in maternity care. In fact, influencing both boys and girls positively on male nurses should be the end goal for the call for more men to get into nursing. The aim is obviously to encourage more boys and men to join nursing. But for the girls, the aim will be to let them know there is nothing wrong with boys wanting to become nurses.

Break those gender stereotypes in both genders while they are still young. Let us raise a generation where young children can look up to nurses simply because they do a great job and not because of their gender. It will hurt no one if a young girl looks up to a male nurse and vice versa.

Chapter 11: Being Part of a Profession Where Women Dominate

Female nurses dominate the nursing profession in terms of numbers. This has created a stereotype that male nurses do not belong in the nursing profession - more so that they aren't cut out for it. Yes, we agree that there are a lot of valuable insights that female nurses have curated over the years. We do not discount their contributions at all. However, we need to be real! Not allowing male nurses to be a part of the nursing team results in a complete inability for high-quality patient care to be realistically achieved.

The number of men in the nursing field has tripled compared to that of the early '70s. And yes, that is all good and well, but is a triple in numbers that significant given that the number of male nurses present was small, to begin with?

Yes, it is great that the number is increasing, but what is stopping more young males from entering nursing? We've discussed the main points in previous chapters, but what about female nurses deterring male nurses from entering the field?

It is one thing for young men to be allowed the opportunity to become male nurses, but are female nurses welcoming men with open arms into the profession? Many would say yes, but in actual fact, male nurses can feel rather overwhelmed. Male nurses may feel that they are being cushioned as they move into nursing. This is actually a good thing!

As men, we are used to being reprimanded when we fail a new task, even if it is the first time. However, female nurses provide an environment conducive to learning, allowing male nurses to hone their skills. They do away with the typical "see one, do one, teach one" mentality, supporting you until you are comfortable with doing the procedure alone. Female nurses understand that learning takes time, and they offer this environment to male nurses that may never have been placed in one that is as uniquely nurturing as the nursing one.

All men are not the same. Yes, we may share some traits, but our values and personalities are different. Some male nurses may be comfortable fighting the status quo, where women dominate nursing. Others may feel they just want to go with the flow. There are ways for both these types of male nurses to feel accepted in the nursing field, and from what we know, although some female nurses are against the idea, 90% of them will create an environment that promotes the growth and development of competent male nurses.

For the 10% that feel that not having male nurses in the field is beneficial, their reasons extend from an already prominent pay gap and losing yet another profession to male domination.

For a young man reading this, let us explain a bit more. It is statistically proven that male nurses, despite being in the minority, are paid more than female nurses. Furthermore, some females fear that male nurses will come to dominate their field. They feel that men already dominate other professions and want to be given a chance to be given a profession that they can call their own. Although this is not progressive, luckily, just a small portion of female nurses feel this way.

Male nurses with a passion for the field should not feel that they cannot make a difference here. Yes, females may have been in the profession for longer, but don't undermine your abilities to change the face of healthcare as a male nurse! As a male nurse, you will be providing a perspective in meetings that won't be attainable by female nurses because, well, they aren't male. This not only promotes critical thinking but also ensures that male nurses are valued enough that they are willing to motivate other young men to enter the nursing profession.

Anyone will work harder should they feel valued. Yes, although mental health may not be as physically evident in males, it does not necessarily mean that they do not have mental health issues. For one, the open and caring nature of women, in general, may promote the bettering of the intrinsic health of many male nurses.

How? Well, it will allow them to talk about what bothers them in a safe environment and where they do not feel their masculinity will be challenged by other men. Although there are some things that only men can say to other men, sometimes the listening ear of a woman can provide a much-needed perspective.

Ultimately, one can see that there is a need for male nurses within a women-dominated field. There is a marked need for a male perspective within the nursing field that will help to improve patient outcomes and create a more diversified profession. Men have an essential role to play, and this needs to be recognized by everyone currently a part of the nursing profession. For young men who want to follow the nursing career path, we need to ensure that they are given the platform to achieve their hopes, dreams, and aspirations. The first step to this is for female nurses to acknowledge that a man's passion for nursing has placed him in the profession, not his need to dominate it.

While there will be some men who would want to dominate the field, the reality is that most male nurses want to care for patients without their gender becoming a major part of their identity. They want to be seen for what they do, not what their gender is.

Being part of a female-dominated profession also means not getting the opportunity to learn some additional skills needed for the career since few people in power relate to your struggles. For example, male nurses will often never receive guidance on how to go about making an intimate touch toward a patient. Male nurses are incredibly vulnerable when it comes to the personal touch, especially with a woman.

While this concern is documented in nursing literature, many critical nursing fundamentals never consider it, probably because such fundamentals are written under the belief that only women are getting into the profession. Yet, it is crucial that male nurses understand just what it takes to provide an intimate touch to a patient without coming off as a pervert. With no guidance on how to go about such things, a male nurse can become stuck or end up in a delicate situation that was not of their own making.

So, it is crucial that there are additions in the nursing syllabus that guide male nurses on how to provide intimate care for female patients without coming off as perverts or putting themselves at risk of getting accused of sexual assault. The most basic of this will often be to ask for permission, but the syllabus needs to be detailed in guiding the male nurses on where and how to go about the process, just as it is for women.

Many male nurses will often be thrilled when they find female nurses who do not view them with suspicion or fear. As with anyone else in a job where they are the minority, they want to feel welcomed and appreciated. They are there to perform their responsibilities and nothing else. No, they are not there to dominate. In fact, while the number of men in nursing is increasing with each passing year, the wealth of opportunities in the field is still very much open to women. So, nursing will remain a female-dominated field for the foreseeable future. Any fear of men dominating the field is greatly unfounded. However, male nurses entering the field will often be full of confidence, and this could make some female nurses feel intimidated. Perhaps that could be why some will think men want to dominate.

There should, thus, be an effort to make some amendments to nursing education to accommodate the new perspective and unique way of caring that male nurses use. For example, as we saw in the last chapter, male nurses often use humor to care. Such small details can be put into consideration to make male nurses feel a lot more welcomed in the profession they love.

They may be the minorities, but male nurses are becoming an essential part of nursing once again, and accommodating them is a win for everyone; female nurses, male nurses themselves, and of course, the whole healthcare sector.

Chapter 12: Coping With Coworker Issues

Working solo is, unfortunately, not how the nursing profession works. With nursing being one of the more team-oriented professions, you need to remember that you aren't just going to be interacting with other nurses. You are a part of a multi-disciplinary team! This means that you will be working with doctors, surgeons, occupational therapists, and other medical personnel to cure a patient holistically.

As life continues, it is just a fact that we won't get along with everyone. This means that you might be in a situation where bickering with another colleague due to differences in the proposed care of a patient may actually harm the patient's health. Now, this does not mean that you can't have misunderstandings with your coworkers, but there is a way to deal with these issues healthily. Also, having an unpleasant interaction with a coworker can completely ruin your mental health and how you provide care to others. The latter is doing a disservice to your patients as a male nurse.

However, to cope with a problematic coworker, you need to know how to identify one. This can be difficult for a male nurse because men don't typically look for issues with others as much as female nurses do.

Yes, that sounds horrible, but if society has taught us anything, gossiping is statistically more common between women than men. When looking at research conducted here in the United States of

America, four of every five female nurses have participated in gossiping about coworkers.

But even though gossiping creates the potential for coworker issues, there are a few more traits and difficulties that the picture-perfect 'difficult coworker' may create. They are as follows:

- Instead of focusing on their work, they would rather create unnecessary drama. This can be anything from telling a bunch of people what another coworker did during the weekend or merely bashing another coworker when not prompted at all.

- Bringing personal problems to work impedes your ability to think and act professionally. Difficult coworkers find it challenging to distinguish between which of their feelings can be expressed in the workplace and which are best kept to themself.

- Not performing their required duties and passing them off to others does not make for happy coworkers. Nurses are already swamped with their own work, and having to pick up someone else's slack will definitely not end well. You really don't want your work being the deciding factor between a colleague finishing up on time or needing to do overtime (and often without compensation).

- Another important coworker issue is the feeling of superiority based on experience. As soon as you start to undermine others and others notice this, you can almost be assured that a dispute will pop up at some point!

As a male nurse, you will meet a myriad of difficult coworkers, even those that deviate a bit from the personalities and actions discussed above. But, you need to be able to deal with these colleagues and not allow them to impede the quality and safety of care that you provide your patients.

So, how do you do that?

If you do not like drama, you need to be able to communicate honestly with your coworker in a private space. You want to make them see how their behavior affects you, but you must also show that you are trying to understand where they are coming from. The last thing you want to be perceived as, especially as a male nurse, is being insensitive.

You want to assume objectively but also ask for feedback from other coworkers. Many others may have had the same issues with a specific coworker and could have devised a way to deal with them and their outbursts. As a male nurse you may want to heed their advice but be mindful that this advice doesn't develop into a gossiping session!

If you have tried absolutely everything and there has been no improvement, it may be time to speak to your superior. You want to show your superior that you at least tried to remedy the situation with your coworker before running to them for assistance. You don't want to be known as someone who complains immediately and looks for solutions later.

If the problems with the said co-worker persist, you can also talk to the supervisor or hospital superintendent. Document the co-worker's persistent issues with you and then forward them to a senior to help resolve them. If push comes to shove, you can even ask them to shift you to another team if the coworker is a part of your team. If they are not, you can then limit your interactions with them. You might find that you can deal better with such a coworker in small doses, so choose that instead of fighting back.

Focus on the good

As that goes on, focus more on the positive relationships you have built. Not everyone will be adversarial to you at the workplace, and not everyone will have a problem with your gender. So, focus more on nurturing those positive relationships and spend more time with people who make your day at work much easier. You cannot change problematic coworkers, but you definitely change the coworkers that you hang around.

You can and should stand up for yourself, but remember not to create a situation where the fact that you are a man can be used against you. For example, if the coworker who has issues with you is female, trying to confront them when they are alone might create more ground for them to create new problems for you.

Even when you talk to them privately, ensure that it is in a public place where nothing can be used against you. Becoming physically aggressive with a coworker also will not help beat the stereotype of men being too aggressive for nursing.

As a male nurse, it is crucial that you take time to understand why your co-worker is acting the way they are. If they are acting mean towards you, try to find out if it is related to something you did. If they are simply looking down on you because of your gender, then you will have no option but to try to avoid them as much as possible. You cannot change a person's way of thinking. That is a choice only they can make.

Positive relationships in the nursing profession are crucial because this is one of the places where working well with a team is vital for your long-term survival. Thus, being someone who has excellent conflict-resolution skills gives you an edge. You do not need to get along with each of your co-workers, but you will definitely need to know how to work with them or how to work well, regardless of their presence.

Remember, while having a good social circle at work is essential, your first order of business at the facility is to work. So, when having problems with a co-worker, just put your head down and keep working. Ultimately, the right people will gravitate toward you and become your friends.

Dealing with difficult coworkers is not easy, especially when you constantly need to work as a part of a team. It may be difficult, especially given that male nurses aren't necessarily primed to voice their opinions when uncomfortable.

However, being put in these situations is how you learn more about dealing with difficult coworkers and growing your professional aptitude as a result! The key is not to let difficult colleagues ruin your day or interfere with the care you provide your patients.

Chapter 13: Why Are They Called Male Nurses?

Many find it rather weird that a man who watches football, dreams about fast cars, has a full-blown beard, and spends hours upon hours at the gym, wants to become a nurse. Rightfully so, put a 'male' into the profession of a nurse, then they would logically be known as a 'male nurse.' But have there been any other names that male nurses have been called?

Well, as soon as you type 'male nurse' into any search bar online, you are not only met with a rather extensive list of jokes about male nurses but also an array of different names for them, which are as creative as a 'murse,' as original as a 'mister sister,' and as simple as 'nurse.' The next question that automatically pops into our minds is why people feel the need to specify whether a nurse is male or female.

Do they not perform the same job and have the same qualifications? They do, but stereotypically they are viewed as being different. When a man chooses nursing, society tends to place them in a state where they are considered less masculine than other men. This view is then perpetuated by continuously referring to men who are nurses as 'male nurses' because it continues to look at them as an anomaly in the profession. Rather than making them feel welcome, it makes it pretty clear to the men that they are in the wrong place.

Historically, a female nurse has been referred to as a 'sister' because of the same degree of caring and nurturing that a sister and nurse share. But just putting a mister in front of 'sister' perpetuates the cycle that male nurses cannot operate and function without being viewed through a female lens.

Polls on social media, as well as results of research studies, feel that there shouldn't be any distinction between male and female nurses. Male nurses have reversed the situation within the role of firefighters. If people referred to women within the profession as 'female firefighters,' it creates double standards, which many females would contest.

If you have the skill, aptitude, knowledge, and motives needed to become a nurse, that is how you should be referred to as. It does not matter whether you are a male or female nurse because both sides are equipped to perform optimally within the medical field. The only time where the gender of the nurse should come into play is when there is a special request by a patient based on religious reasons, personal modesty, or any of the other reasons previously discussed.

The term 'male nurse' is unfortunately not going to disappear spontaneously. The public and other nurses have felt the need to establish the difference between a male and a female nurse. By respectfully reminding others that just because you are a male nurse does not mean you are less or more qualified to perform the same occupation, the gender affiliation can be removed, and the nursing profession can move forward to achieve its true potential.

On the other end, it is also crucial that men in nursing also stop making their gender part of their identity at work, even if it comes with some 'celebrity status.'

Indeed, while most of the harm comes from the outside and others within the field, some men who have taken up nursing are using their gender identity to earn celebrity status when in the field. As minorities in the field, men will stand out and be looked at with curiosity, envy, admiration, and disdain. This attention will often make many men uncomfortable, but some who crave celebrity status will embrace this.

Thus, such men will openly and gladly accept the title 'male nurse' and could even use it as part of their job description. This might seem like them embracing their job, and I am sure many of them do. But what it does is that it pushes back against the efforts that others in the field are making toward making nurses less tied to gender.

We need more men to get into nursing, and they need to see and know of men in nursing who are proud of their work. However, continually referring to men in nursing as male nurses means these young boys will simply inherit the view that men in nursing are such a sight to behold that they need to be gendered to avoid confusion.

We Are Headed in the Right Direction

Many male nurses in the field are changing the perception of men in nursing and are turning attention away from the phrase 'male nurse' to simply becoming 'nurse.' Many men in nursing, for example, are campaigning against other male nurses from referring to them using the term.

There are many forums and campaigns in the profession which aim to encourage more men to get into nursing. These drives will often target students in nursing, aiming to bring them into the field. However, many are moving away from referring to themselves as 'male nurses' and instead simply encouraging more men to join the profession. They believe that the label 'male nurse' creates a negative distinction for men.

Thus, even in situations where men embrace the celebrity status of being a 'male nurse,' dropping the word 'male' and simply referring to themselves as 'nurse' goes a long way in fighting the stereotypes than making "male nurse" an identity.

In modern times, many men who get into nursing proudly call themselves nurses and do not need the term male added in front to affirm to them that they are still masculine. This is, by far, the most significant step in the right direction towards dropping the distinction of male/female nurse and instead making it the norm for any gender to enter the field.

These men understand that when people in the profession are separated into gendered categories, then the stereotypes that come with them mean that there will be fewer collaborations at the workplace, which might lead to friction between genders and make it harder for everyone in the field.

Female nurses have also jumped on the bandwagon of stopping the distinction between male/female nurses at work. They understand that when at work, everyone contributes to the work environment, and thus, the less separation there is based on superficial things such as gender, the best it is for everyone.

Chapter 14: Male Nurses Balance the Nursing Profession

Logically thinking, there are many things that a male can explain that a female can struggle to comprehend, and vice versa. Regardless, male nurses are needed in the profession; there is no doubt about that!

It is a known fact that as one creates an environment where males and females perform the same jobs, it encourages critical thinking and enables the profession to move forward as a whole. In order to balance out the nursing profession, stereotypes need to be broken.

It needs to be emphasized that male nurses work just as hard as female nurses and that their gender has absolutely nothing to do with their ability to care for a patient. Male nurses can fill the gap where female nurses struggle, especially when it comes to lifting patients from their beds to a chair for mobilization or moving around heavy equipment.

The same is true for when male nurses may struggle with being too forthright. In contrast, female nurses can teach them how to be more understanding and compassionate when delivering bad news or dealing with a patient whose emotions are in disarray.

Rasmussen University did a study where male nurses were asked whether they felt their presence established a more balanced profession. Many agreed but noted marked differences in how men and women think differently and approach the same tasks from different angles and mindsets.

However, many felt that male nurses are now sensitized to the gender disparity within the nursing profession. For male nurses to balance their careers, they need not perceive every male-based characteristic pointed out by a female colleague as an attack on them being a man. Not everything is an attack on your professional integrity!

However, male nurses take an immense amount of pride in their job. Every time they are mistaken for a more 'male-presumed' role, such as a doctor or pharmacist, redirecting somebody else's thoughts to the realization that men can be nurses has a broad knock-on effect. By changing the perspectives of those not used to the presence of male nurses, you are allowing them to see the possibilities of it, leading to them not shooting down the idea that they or their own children can enter the profession. This is how one can establish a true balance of numbers in nursing.

Male nurses are changing the perception that gender characteristics and the prevailing public image of men stop them from making good nurses. While many men will choose nursing for practical reasons; higher salary, more job opportunities, job security, or working conditions, a similarly large number of men also prefer the profession due to altruistic desires. Whatever the case, as long as the men entering the field are the best, their presence helps provide a balanced look to the nursing profession.

A Different Perspective

Men show a unique perspective and depth to the nursing profession. This is not just how they are wired to think but also the way they deal with emotions. They create a well-rounded team that benefits any patient they interact with. The approaches of a man and woman towards care are different; thus, having both genders at work means that the patients receive care from two different perspectives, all working towards the same goal.

This makes the patient's recovery faster and much more wholesome. For example, women will care for a patient by providing physical touch, while men show they care through banter and shared laughter from time to time. Both of these approaches to nursing are crucial and help the patient recover better, hence why men are needed to balance the profession for the best of the patients.

Therefore, we need more nurses who embody the best characteristics of the profession regardless of gender and fewer nurses who got their break into the profession simply because they are female.

Just because someone is female does not mean they will make a great nurse, and just because someone is male does not mean they will be a terrible nurse. We need to change the perception of male nurses from within, and the rest of society will catch up.

Chapter 15: Are Male Nurses Happier Than Female Nurses?

When looking at whether male nurses are happier than female nurses, many different avenues can be taken to deduce this, not to mention the various domains of human beings that are influenced by happiness. So, we'll first look at the emotions a male nurse feels while on the job.

When a male nurse feels appreciated in the role that he is in, naturally, he will be happier than if he was treated differently from other nurses. Yes, male nurses are a rare breed, but they have the same qualifications as any other nurse and should not be treated differently based on being male.

Thankfully, male nurses are often valued for going against the status quo and following their dreams that are based on a passion for being selflessly involved in a patient's journey.

When we look at what makes a man happy, one of the central answers is their family. More often than not, a man feels obliged to be the breadwinner of their family and to be able to provide for all of his family's needs financially. Naturally, a man would want to be able to enjoy his work whilst being afforded the opportunity to spend time with his family.

Professions in healthcare are notorious for taking so much time from people that living everyday family-focused life is deemed near impossible. However, the **flexibility of schedules** that nurses have, especially those who choose the route of a travel nurse, affords the opportunity to really strike that perfect balance between being a family man and a professional nurse. By asking any family man what makes him sleep with a smile on his face, one of the more common answers would be knowing that his family is safe and has all they need.

Another prime point of happiness for men is **receiving praise** from other professionals and even their patients. Society dictates that men 'do not' need as much credit when doing a good job. This is entirely false!

Are men also not human?

Do they not also want to know that they are doing a good job?

Of course, they do! Tell a male nurse that he handled that case well or performed that cannula insertion beautifully; true, they may not show their happiness physically. Still, their emotional domain is beaming with pride and satisfaction! Many female nurses base their performance on how well others perceive their skill sets. This is true for male nurses, but men are better at hiding their emotions than females. This is why when a male nurse shows their happiness just know that it is genuine and heartfelt.

Male nurses are more likely to be happier than female nurses as their presence within the profession is already **altering preconceived notions** about nursing. Being able to see how this growth is influencing other young men to venture into the nursing profession will allow male nurses to beam with pride. This could even be to the extent that they have a higher degree of job satisfaction as they are inadvertently (or directly) changing the functioning of the nursing profession whilst shaping the mindsets of younger generations of men.

The Revolution

Indeed, the fact that they are **trailblazers** in the field means that they take great pride in being the people who are leading a kind of 'revolution.' This sense of pride comes from the greater sense of purpose courtesy of being the people breaking gender stereotypes.

Male nurses cease to be just nurses, but they also become role models, people who others are looking up to shape their path in nursing. This greater sense of purpose can also contribute to male nurses being happier than female nurses.

Another reason could be that men receive **higher pay** on average in nursing. Since male nurses will often take on additional responsibilities aside from their primary nursing assignments, such as lifting heavy equipment or taking on late-night shifts, they receive higher pay on average. Better pay makes male nurses feel much more welcomed and appreciated in the profession.

The beauty of nursing is that you work directly with people, and being in a position to nurture people back to full health is probably the most **fulfilling** part of the job. For men in particular, since there have been few male nurses in recent history, male nurses could be finding more joy in nursing because it is a novelty to them. Perhaps female nurses might have become desensitized to the job a little.

But for male nurses, since they need to work twice as hard to get into the profession in the first place, the joy of getting their job done and doing it well is unrivaled and is seen as the perfect culmination of the years of struggle through nursing school. This could be another reason male nurses are happier than their female counterparts.

That said, it should be noted that both male and female nurses will need to come together and work for a better work environment for all nurses so that all categories of nurses are happy at the workplace. While better pay will make male nurses happier, if the income is believed to be unfair by female nurses, it can lead to strains at the workplace, and the joy of the male nurse at work will be short-lived.

So, male nurses should ensure that the joy that they feel in the profession is shared along with the female nurses so that everyone at the workplace is satisfied and contented with their job.

People in authority should use the enthusiasm and bliss of male nurses to further make the profession an excellent place for people with a passion for it. Male nurses can be a great way of helping bring back more people into the nursing profession, both men and women!

Chapter 16: Nursing is Not Just for Women

When we were young, we often thought of nursing as a job strictly for women. But when we grew up, we realized that nursing is a job that both genders can and should do. The more men get into nursing, the better it is for everyone in society; this is down to various reasons.

Now, while the prevailing attitude towards male nurses from the larger society is negative, a study conducted by the American Sociological Association found that most female nurses welcomed their male counterparts. In fact, many female nurses felt that more men needed to be encouraged to join the field. This is good news because it means that many female nurses are willing to work with men, making it easier for men to work in the field even when they do not have a male counterpart in a facility.

And the welcoming nature of female nurses is down to several reasons. First, the more nurses, the better it is for everyone. Nurses are a critical part of medical care. They are the line of contact with patients in most cases and, thus, will often need to be more to fulfill this purpose well. The more nurses, the better care patients receive, and the less fatigue nurses will have by taking care of more patients than they usually would.

The U.S Bureau of Labor and Statistics states that over one million registered nurses are set to retire by the end of 2022. And while the employment of nurses is set to go up, unfortunately, the number of people looking for jobs in the field is not rising fast enough. Therefore, it does not matter whether a nurse is male or female; as long as they pass the qualifications, they should work in the field to help cope with the projected increase in demand for nurses. Female nurses, then, view male nurses as crucial to helping fill the gap and, thus, are more open to welcoming them into the field if it means more shared responsibilities.

The Prevailing Problem

Male nurses play a critical role in advancing the nursing field due to breaking down gender stereotypes in the field. Most gender stereotypes view nursing as a feminine job and being a doctor as a masculine job in healthcare. The belief is that men should become doctors and women nurses. Thus, to these people, a man becoming a nurse is a sign of failure for that man and masculinity.

Indeed, such gender stereotypes around nursing are often perpetuated by lazy TV writing, which often portrays male nurses as either being effeminate (coding for them being either gay or queer) or comical (meaning that they cannot be taken seriously, with the joke often coming at the expense of them being a nurse).

Thus, when we have more male nurses practicing, not only do they help in providing patient care, but they also help in creating positive perceptions of men in nursing. This means that many more boys in the future will want to become nurses and be proud of that choice and that society will begin to view nursing as the critical field in healthcare that it is.

As we have seen, the negative view of male nurses often does not come from female nurses but from the outside world. Even patients admitted to hospitals are welcoming of male nurses, and some even prefer them to female nurses. By breaking down these stereotypes, more boys will feel a lot more comfortable and confident in saying that nursing is something that they would like to do without being judged for it, either considered too weak for 'manly jobs' or considered homosexual.

Another reason why more male nurses are needed is that working alongside female nurses can help improve patient care and advocate for better policies and practices. Let's be honest; the society we live in now is often more inclined to listen to men than women. Thus, male nurses can bring in that instrumental male voice that helps improve the healthcare field, not just for themselves but also for other female nurses.

This situation is not ideal, and nursing needs to compensate nurses better regardless of gender. Still, male nurses help bring much-needed positive outlook and respect to the field.

Male nurses' presence in the nursing field also helps improve their careers both in compensation and work environments. Remember, despite being the minority, most male nurses receive, on average, higher salaries than their female counterparts. With their pay higher, there will also be the net effect of increased pay for the female nurses, especially those who have been in the field for a long time. Male nurses can also use their voices to back female nurses in asking for better pay, especially when the roles performed are all similar.

Another reason why male nurses are needed is that they take away the burden of caring for male patients from female nurses. Intimate care could open up the potential for sexual abuse if a nurse of the opposite gender does it for another. This is why male nurses are also discouraged from taking up duties such as changing diapers, dressing, cleaning private parts, or bathing female patients. The same is true for female nurses. Thus, with male nurses in the picture, female nurses can be tasked with providing such intimate care for female patients while male nurses do the same for male patients.

Did you know that nursing was not traditionally a female-dominated field as it is now and that many of the barriers male nurses face now started less than 200 years ago? Indeed, before that, men were considered primary caregivers for sick patients. Men were the primary caregivers as far back as Ancient Rome, and were the primary caregivers in the Black Plague of 300 AD and nursed the injured during major events before the 1900s.

While it is all great to have more men in nursing, let us look at some barriers that male nurses face:

Barriers Male Nurses Face

The biggest barrier, gender stereotypes, began some 150-160 years ago. Florence Nightingale, considered the mother of modern nursing, did a stellar job during the Crimean War when she treated injured soldiers and trained other nurses while at it. However, she perpetuated the myth that men could not make good nurses because their hands were 'hard and horny' and that caring and nurturing occurred effortlessly for women. Thus, during the 1850s, when she set up formal nursing in the UK, she worked with only female nurses. And as the UK spread its influence worldwide, this way of nursing was duplicated.

This is what has shaped the **common public perception** that men are simply not suitable to be nurses, no matter how caring and nurturing they are. This perception has been perpetuated in American pop culture by TV shows and movies which, as mentioned, treat male nurses either as being gay or as a joke. The perception is that nursing is not 'male enough' for young men and that even if a man chooses to pursue it, it is not their first choice. Thus, it is not surprising, then, that many career advisors do not endorse nursing to boys when they are in high school. The truth is that many men who pursue nursing will often have a very close influence on that career path, perhaps having someone close to them be in the field.

Then there is also the fact that male nurses tend **not to have access to male role models** during their training and their entry into the practice. The lack of access to male nurses to look up to makes it even more challenging for the male nurse in an environment where they are made to feel as though they do not belong. This can lead to professional isolation, where the man is unable to build work relationships that can help them enter the nursing field as smoothly as possible.

In most cases, many female nurses are welcoming of male nurses and are often eager to work with them as they come into the field. Even then, we still know that the presence of someone you can relate to when in a new environment is crucial. Think of how women who join male-dominated fields also feel isolated no matter how welcoming their male counterparts are. A diverse set of genders in the nursing field, just like in any other field, helps not only in providing better care for patients, it helps male nurses have someone they can relate to and look up to

Additionally, **not every female nurse is welcoming** to male nurses. Remember, society still views male nurses as an anomaly; thus, some female nurses will bear these perceptions when at work, thus, making them less trusting of their male counterparts and dissociating from them.

Another barrier is often more **institutional**. Due to the prevailing belief that nursing is for women, most examinations are written with female nursing students in mind. A study that was done by Kiekkas et al. (2016) found that male nurses were often on the wrong end of gender bias when it came to written examinations.

This becomes even worse when we consider clinical practice requirements. Different standards were applied to the students based on gender differences. This barrier is perhaps one of the biggest hurdles that any male nurse can face. When the thing that is supposed to make you a nurse is designed around stereotypes, then it becomes even harder for you to qualify to enter the field. It is no surprise then that male nurses make up a large percentage of the 25 percent of student nurses who drop out before completion.

Another gender stereotype around male nurses is that since they are men, they can be subject to heavier manual work or be tasked with taking care of the most aggressive and violent patients without needing much else. While men are generally larger and stronger than women, male nurses choose the field because they want to care for and nurture patients and not simply be thrust into situations where they have to deal with the most aggressive patients daily.

Another barrier that male nurses need to overcome is the barrier of their own thoughts. While it does take great mental fortitude to stay in nursing school, graduate, and then join the workforce, many male nurses soon begin to feel strained and stressed once they are on the job.

Often, this comes down to the fact that they may not have another male nurse to associate with, but it could also be that the nurse begins to actually understand the reality of being a male nurse. These stressful thoughts can cause a male nurse to head on a downward spiral; thus, it is crucial to get integrated into a group to help them deal with the stresses of the job. The American Association of Men in Nursing (AAMN), for example, is a group that supports men who are nurses in several capacities. Not only does the association provide you with access to opportunities in the nursing profession, but it also offers support and guidance to male nurses. Such an association helps male nurses overcome their own mental barriers and get down to working in nursing.

So, on top of the daily challenges of being a nurse, male nurses also have to deal with specific challenges simply because they are men working in a field that is still perceived as mostly for women. It is no wonder that many female nurses are welcoming of their male counterparts.

Can We All Get along?

As mentioned, while many female nurses are welcoming of male nurses, there are still questions as to whether, in the long term, male and female nurses can get along. The reality is that there will definitely be a lot of challenges for male and female nurses to get along. Still, ultimately, the realization that we are all working toward the same goal should help us work better together.

Nursing is a field that many of us consider a calling. This means that you chose the field due to the desire to care for and be of service to others. Thus, with this in mind, both male and female nurses can work easier and better together. Healthcare facilities benefit when patients are well taken care of and fully recovered due to the efforts nurses put into the tasks. Plus, having both male and female nurses makes the job easier when it's time to care for patients of different sexes.

Getting along also helps in making communication easier. Aside from scientific knowledge, nursing requires you to learn how to communicate effectively with colleagues and patients. Both male and female nurses need to be able to speak freely and openly with each other for various reasons. First, the transfer of knowledge and experience happens in this way.

Secondly, communication helps break down assumptions and stereotypes that one may be having about the other, allowing for much better relations at work. Then there is also the fact that communication helps reduce the male nurse's professional isolation. Oftentimes, a male nurse can find himself as the only male nurse in a facility of several female nurses. Without proper communication, this nurse can easily become isolated and unable to do much work. Communication also helps the nurses organize and coordinate their care activities for the betterment of the patient.

Another reason why male and female nurses need to get along is for their own health. Nursing is a stressful field and becomes even more stressful during major health emergencies like disasters, disease outbreaks, and pandemics. Thus, both male and female nurses communicating openly helps them build better work relationships and, therefore, work better and easier with the patients.

Embracing the Differences

The different outlooks on things between men and women can often mean that it is a bit challenging for male and female nurses to get along. The reason why this is an issue for nurses and not others in the healthcare field like doctors is that nursing is a lot more collaborative on a daily basis. As a nurse, you will need to work with others each day. Therefore, the more male nurses get into the field, the more the different ways of looking at things become evident.

However, many female nurses have embraced the differences between the two genders and are welcoming of men for precisely these differences.

The first is that men bring calm to the profession. Now, this is not to say that female nurses are volatile. After all, being patient and calm is a necessary part of becoming a nurse. But the reality is, based on what they went through, male nurses will often be a lot more accepting and calm, which is why they are in the field despite the prevailing stereotypes around them choosing to pursue nursing as a profession.

Picture sitting through years of nursing school, studying for examinations, while also fighting against gender stereotypes (both individual and institutional), graduating, and then joining the nursing field. All these are marks that the male nurses who graduate and enter the nursing workforce are people who are incredibly calm, composed, and patient, probably a lot more than an ordinary person would be.

Their fight against gender stereotypes means they learn how to be level-headed even under extreme work-related stress because they had encountered stressful situations before and emerged victorious.

Another difference is the fact that male nurses earn promotions faster than female nurses. While this might seem unfair, it often comes down to a major factor that most men possess – confidence. For male nurses to remain steadfast in their choice to pursue nursing amidst frowns from all corners of society, they need to have very high levels of confidence. And it is this confidence that is the reason why most male nurses gain promotion faster than women.

Male nurses possess that intangible quality of being able to do what they want to do and doing it to the best of their ability without putting much thought into what people will say. Such confidence and belief in one's abilities mark someone for promotion or a pay rise, and it seems as though male nurses have mastered this, hence why they are considered for promotions and pay raises.

That said, this is a difference that, if not properly dealt with, can result in animosity between male and female nurses. While male nurses will often be more confident than female nurses, the fact that there are more female nurses than male nurses means that there will always be a wider pool of experienced female nurses to choose from compared to male nurses.

Therefore, both male and female nurses should ensure that they work together to get the right people promoted, as it ensures that their career growth is not stalled due to either real or perceived gender biases. Indeed, the way that both male and female nurses have embraced each other in the field means that they can often back the best person for promotion, whether male or female and can use their collective voice in speaking up against promotions they feel are not done on merit.

Male nurses need to embrace themselves and their careers because that is what gives them joy. They should pay lip service to other people's prejudices about them and their work. With additional support from female nurses, men in nursing are guaranteed a good, conducive working environment and fair compensation far better than anything they have presumed.

Chapter 17: Female Nurses' Perspective on Working with Male Nurses

As a female nurse, working with male nurses provides a very different experience from working with fellow female nurses. These experiences will often be both positive and negative. The positive experiences show us how female nurses view male nurses in a positive light and why they are open to working with them. The negative experiences also show us where we can improve, so that male nurses do not become a burden to female nurses as their numbers increase in the field.

So, let us begin with the positive experience of female nurses working with male nurses.

Positive Perception Working with Male Nurses

Male nurses have had a mostly positive impact in healthcare, which is why female nurses are very welcoming of their presence in the field.

Nursing has mostly been a female affair for several decades now, but more men joining the field provides a new and unique experience to female nurses. As a female nurse, working with a male nurse helps open up your perspective on gender roles and why for the most part, they always work to limit all of us from achieving what we need to do.

By breaking down gender barriers, male nurses help female nurses appreciate their job more due to learning of the difficulties and stereotypes that male nurses have had to deal with and continue to deal with as they work.

So, as a female nurse working with a male nurse, you get to understand that men, just like women, can also be nurturing and caring, they can be patient and composed under stress, and they can do any other task that female nurses can do.

Another major advantage of working with male nurses is that they take away some of the burdens that female nurses have had to contend with for years of being the only ones in the field. While female nurses have grown to accept taking care of male patients intimately, the process remains awkward for female nurses. And it becomes even harder for female nurses when they have to deal with patients who might not want a woman to bath them due to cultural or religious reasons. Such patients will even turn down a wipe-down from a female nurse and might even altogether refuse to be washed by the female nurse, thus putting everything on hold.

But it goes even beyond intimate care. Male patients might have unique conditions which another male nurse could only understand in the room. Men will often be coy around women when experiencing conditions that they feel make them look less masculine. This attitude continues even when the man is in a hospital or an emergency situation and can, thus, delay the examination, diagnosis, or treatment process. Thus, male nurses help prevent this male-patient-female-nurse misunderstanding as they help provide better insight to male patients in ways that a female nurse could not.

Male nurses' presence means that male patients will be more open to revealing their conditions since they will feel more open to opening up about their struggles with male nurses. It also means that the diagnosis or examination process is hastened due to the patient becoming more willing to open up.

However, since male nurses are still the minority in the nursing field, such men might often not get their wish, which could result in them reluctantly accepting a female nurse. This situation can make the job harder for the female nurse. Thus, this is why female nurses hold positive perceptions of more men joining the field. It would mean that the patients who prefer male nurses finally get attended to by someone they prefer, rather than having to contend with a nurse they do not want simply because of gender stereotypes.

Furthermore, young male patients will, in particular, find it harder to relate to women most of the time. As already mentioned, boys are often embarrassed about changes to their bodies in front of women. Thus, the male nurse can help them feel much more comfortable speaking about their health issues and make them comfortable throughout their stay in the hospital.

And it goes beyond patients. Female nurses have often had to contend with male doctors dismissing them due to gender barriers that place more emphasis on male voices. Thus, these male doctors will often either treat a female nurse's concerns as trivial overreactions or simply ignore them. But with more male nurses in the field, doctors will listen more to the nurses collectively.

Male nurses' presence in the field has helped the nursing field be taken more seriously by many people in the outside world. As mentioned previously, gender stereotypes mean people look at nursing as a field for people who fail to become doctors. With more women than men in the field, this stereotype has been reinforced, especially since many people believe that only men can and should become doctors.

However, as more men choose to become nurses and make it their first choice, it has forced many people to reconsider their thoughts about nursing. Sure, men who get into nursing are still viewed through narrow lenses of gender stereotypes, but there is a changing belief around nursing and its role in society as more men choose to join the field.

Obviously, it would have been better if nursing had been taken a lot more seriously before. Still, many female nurses look at male nurses as bringing in the much-needed respect for the nursing field that has sorely been lacking over the years.

Male nurses also tend to be a lot more balanced and levelheaded, making them easier to work with. While a calm and patient attitude is necessary for one to get into nursing, for female nursing, other factors such as PMS or pregnancy can cause a change in a woman's body hormones, thus, resulting in changes in attitude and temperament.

However, men tend to be a lot less prone to frequent hormonal changes, and even when they happen, they often don't affect their temperament that much. Thus, unless male nurses experience a significant event in their life, they will often be calm and levelheaded most of the time, even when dealing with stubborn patients or refusing to cooperate. Their levelheadedness can bring a much-needed balance to the nursing sector. They can often be reliably called upon to take over from a nurse struggling with a patient who refuses to cooperate.

Another upside of male nurses is that some do not mind being called in to do some heavy lifting. Now, I understand that this is a gender stereotype that male nurses have to contend with, where they are often tasked with simply doing the heavy lifting around the facility and not much nurturing and caring.

However, most female nurses are often appreciative of having a male nurse whom they can call upon to lift heavy items from time to time. Since, on average, men are larger and stronger than women, they can lift heavier stuff than women can. These could be lifting heavier patients or carrying medical equipment and such. When female nurses need to lift heavy items, it would require them to come together and use their collective strength for the purpose, and this could lead to a shortage of nurses elsewhere.

However, it should be noted that female nurses will often want male nurses to do more of the nursing they are required to as it shares that responsibility across the board. Thus, they will often not resort to calling a male nurse each time they need something moved, or a patient lifted.

Therefore, male nurses should not view this as female nurses seeing them as muscles only and nothing more. Rather, their masculine strength can be a convenience from time to time when things get a little too heavy.

Male nurses, despite still being the minority and stereotyped, are still considered crucial in helping improve the working environment in nursing. The society that we live in is largely patriarchal. This means that many people in power are often men, and these men will listen more to other men than women. Thus, female nurses view male nurses as a necessary addition to the field as they help amplify the voices of the nurses to the relevant authorities, whether it be with regard to payment, work environment, or any other crucial concerns in the nursing environment.

Regarding promotions, prevailing evidence shows that more male nurses often get promoted. However, from a female nurse perspective, male nurses can use their influence to also front other female nurses for promotions since their voice, despite being in the minority, still has sway over the people in power. Thus, for female nurses, male nurses can help them gain promotions by backing them up, especially through vocal advocacy.

A 2022 Nurse Salary Research Report showed that nurses had seen their pay rise significantly across the U.S, which comes at a period when male nurses continue to join the field. This is good news for any student who is getting into the nursing field. Nurse salary concerns are often more likely to be listened to and acted upon faster when more men get into the field. So, from a female nurse's perspective, having more male nurses helps improve the whole nursing sector for everyone.

Working with male nurses also means they will often be more open to overtime, thus lifting the burden from female nurses. A 2017 Medscape RN/LPN Compensation Report found that male nurses tended to work more overtime than women. This means that male nurses will often take on a lot more responsibilities or work with those late-night emergencies that demand a lot from healthcare workers. For example, due to their physical strength, they will often do much of the heavy lifting in the hospital. They also tended to gravitate towards positions that paid them hourly rather than salaried. Thus, they opted to work more hours to increase their pay.

So, female nurses appreciate that this could help balance the work hours and allow them to go home earlier or take on other responsibilities which they would be more willing to take, such as attending outpatients.

Many female nurses view working with male nurses as coming with several benefits beyond simply the fact that they add up numbers to the nursing sector.

However, as with many things, female nurses do not have only a positive perspective working with male nurses.

Negative Perception Working with Male Nurses

Let us begin with the fact that, while many female nurses welcome male nurses as they help in increasing numbers in the field, other female nurses would still very much prefer that women continue getting hired.

This is because, for long, nursing has become something of a women's domain, a place where many women can call their own. Thus, to them, the addition of men in this field ruins this whole view. These female nurses then see men getting into nursing as **men taking over a space that was simply there for women**. To them, rather than view male nurses entering the field as further proof of the fight against gendered stereotypes, they see it as a continuation of 'male dominance' into a field that women have made their own.

But, as we have seen, nursing was initially a male-only domain long before the 20th century, and thus, having men in the field is simply a way of improving healthcare for everyone by choosing the best people for the job regardless of gender. However, this negative perception from female nurses means that to them, gender needs to be a factor and only women should be trained and hired into the field. They view male nurses more as competitions rather than colleagues there to help make the healthcare sector a better place.

However, note that such thoughts from nurses are infrequent and that most nurses are open to more men entering the field.

But a perspective that is quite common is that **male nurses could do better than nursing**. Male nurses are indeed welcome by female nurses, but the view that men make doctors and women make nurses still persists at the depths of many female nurses' points of view. So, while outwardly, the nurse will be open to working with and even becoming friends with the male nurse, at the back of their mind, they will often wonder if the male nurse could have done better and perhaps become something else in healthcare.

This is no fault of the nurses who think like this. Society is still grappling with the reality that men can and are taking on nurturing and caring jobs. Thus, even when nurses go through training, learn about nursing and get into healthcare, understand that male nurses are also a thing, they still will have that negative view of male nurses at the back of their minds. Luckily, this perspective is one of the easiest to change.

As long as a female nurse is welcoming to their male counterpart, open to working with them, and is not actively hostile towards them, she can easily overcome this negative view of the male nurse.

While male nurses are caring and nurturing, there is still the perception among female nurses that they are **not as caring as female nurses are**. Once again, this perspective is shaped by how society views men and their ability to nurture. Men are seen as less caring, less nurturing, and less emotionally intelligent than women, and this view is held firmly by some of the female nurses in the field.

Thus, such female nurses will tend to be less trusting of the male nurse, believing that they are incapable of showing empathy and that if they do, then they are pretending. So, suppose they are in a position of power. In that case, such nurses will often not assign the male nurse any duties to care for and nurture patients and will, instead, use the male nurse as a handyman whose only job is to lift heavy patients and equipment around the hospital setting.

This view towards male nurses is sexist and could be a significant reason male nurses can have difficulty integrating into the workforce after completing their studies. The suspicion of the male nurses will mean that the female nurse will not only doubt the male nurse's capacity to care for patients, but it can also translate to animosity towards the male nurse.

Thus, this makes an already awkward situation become hostile and toxic. Considering the fact that we are short of nurses in many parts of the U.S, the last thing would be for male nurses to quit due to frustrations that they encounter at the workplace.

Some female nurses also view male nurses as people who are much **more likely to be creeps** and, thus, need constant supervision or should not attend to patients intimately. There is no doubt that there are male nurses who are creeps and consider nursing an easy way to live out their dark fantasies. And gender stereotypes have made people believe that only men can be creeps; thus, they need to be watched constantly. However, there have also been female nurses who have turned out to be creeps, yet that has not stopped female nurses from working with patients and often without direct supervision unless they carry out medical procedures and need directions.

There will always be people who choose nursing for their own diabolical purposes, but female nurses should not always view all male nurses as people who are there for such intentions. Most people who choose nursing will often be happy and ready to serve others and will work professionally whether or not they are supervised.

Another negative perspective some female nurses have about male nurses is that male nurses will often **be paid a lot more regardless of what they do** and their qualifications. Now, one of the positive perspectives we spoke about was that male nurses helped all nurses earn better in general. However, while nurses make much more in general, male nurses earn more on average than female nurses. This statistic was captured in a 2018 Nursing Salary Research Report which found that male nurses make $6000 a year more than female nurses on average. This disparity in the pay gap, called the gender pay gap, is a major problem, not just in nursing but also in many fields worldwide.

But the negative perception female nurses have that male nurses earn more regardless of qualifications or job done is not true. The 2017 Medscape RN/LPN Compensation report, which found that men were more probable to grind overtime, stated this as one of the reasons they tended to earn more on average. Another reason was that men were also more probable to work in inpatient facilities, which often paid much extra than outpatient facilities.

Furthermore, the study also found that men tended to work more in urban areas than in rural areas compared to female nurses. Again, male nurses were also more likely to negotiate their salaries higher, which was less observed in female nurses. All these factors, then, contribute to the fact that male nurses earn more than female nurses do.

While the **confidence** male nurses bring to the nursing field is necessary, a negative perception that some female nurses may have is **equating this with arrogance**. As we read previously, one of the major reasons why male nurses will often get a lot more promotions and better pay than their female counterparts is their confidence.

This confidence is what makes them more willing to take up more challenging positions, work overtime and take on more challenging responsibilities. This confidence also makes them more willing to negotiate their salaries higher. When male nurses do this, they gain more trust from their employers and many patients and catch the eyes of other nurses around them, who may consider them the best-placed people to take up higher positions.

However, when female nurses feel intimidated by this, they may view the male nurses as arrogant and doing too much. This can cause some resentment to build up and lead to friction in the workplace.

While there is no doubt that there could be some arrogance there, most male nurses will find being in an all-female-unit a bit intimidating and, thus, will often simply want to hit the ground running as soon as possible. To ensure that this happens then, they work extra hard and take on additional responsibilities to win the approval of their colleagues. They will also try to get on good terms with the doctors and other seniors in the hospital to get going faster in the new work environment. This could be why male nurses work overtime and take on more challenges – to show their colleagues that they are fit for the job and are willing to do all that is necessary to keep it.

They will also be a lot more outspoken and willing to ask questions. But because some female nurses feel intimidated by this, they can view this as arrogance. This perception might get even worse when the male nurse has an unwavering belief in themselves and does not show any signs of backing down.

While men can sometimes take their confidence to extreme levels, we need more male nurses to show confidence in themselves for the better of everyone. Male nurses are still working against persistent stereotypes to do something they love; thus, female nurses should not view them as arrogant.

Rather, they should be welcoming of them and help them settle better and faster in the new work environment. When male nurses work in an environment where they feel welcomed and appreciated, they will not even notice that they are working in an all-female unit. They will simply put their head down to work and get used to it.

Settled male nurses in the profession is a win for everyone, and more so for female nurses. There is little reason for female nurses to feel intimidated by the presence of male nurses in the field because women still outnumber men when it comes to joining nursing school and also when it comes to graduating from college. We all need each other in this profession because nurses are in high demand right now.

As the world slowly recovers from the effects of the pandemic, many healthcare workers may have died from the pandemic. Some may have chosen to leave the profession after (either from burnout, stress, or long-term effects of COVID), while others may be heading into retirement (up to 500,000 nurses are going to retire by the end of 2022, according to the U.S Bureau of Labor Statistics).

The American Nurses Association (ANA) projects that the country will need an additional 1.1 million registered nurses to not only replace the nurses leaving the field but also to expand the sector.

Thus, the more female nurses change their negative perception of male nurses, the easier it will be for more nurses to get into the field, including male nurses. If not, the persistent nursing problems could only worsen, with the demand for healthcare increasing as more and more of the aging population require consistent medical care and health complications worsen. Older people now are living much longer and, thus, get to ages where they experience health problems that need constant medical care.

Beat the Perceptions

For the male nurses, most female nurses will be very welcoming of you in the profession. However, these negative perceptions will often come to the fore from time to time since they remain ingrained in many female nurses' psyches. Thus, to avoid letting these perceptions get to you, ensure you do a great job.

There is no better way to change people's negative perception of you than doing the job you are asked to do well and even going beyond. Thus, while you might have a hard time fitting in socially into an all-female unit, the best way to quickly adapt is to do your job well.

Show your caring and nurturing side even when you still feel out of place and feel uncomfortable. Make patients feel comfortable with your presence such that you are the nurse they ask about when you are not around. Make your presence felt by doing a great job to the best of your abilities. This will make your presence felt without you needing to get involved in office politics.

As you consistently do the job well, the female colleagues will have no option but to acknowledge that your presence is actually more helpful than harmful and will begin to embrace you in the facility.

Another way to beat the negative perception female nurses may have towards male nurses is to be an outspoken defendant of female nurses in general. Standing up for your female nurses is a sure way of getting them to trust you and change how they view you and other men in the field.

Remember, while male nurses are a minority in the nursing field, the fact that we live in a patriarchal society means that they will often get more people in authority to listen. To change the view that you are there to take the positions of female nurses, speak up for and defend female nurses. Add your voice to the calls for a better working environment, pay, and maternity leave conditions for female nurses. Even when you do not feel like any of the issues raised by female nurses affect you, join in the fight because when they are comfortable, the whole work environment will be comfortable.

Remember, female nurses still outnumber male nurses in the U.S by 9.5 to 1, and thus, they still make up the majority of the workforce in the field. So, even when something does not directly affect male nurses, it will indirectly affect you. For example, if female nurses face persistent challenges in the work environment that you do not face, this could lower their morale, thus making them more likely to quit.

When they quit, that leads to shortages, and shortages mean more workload for you. Same if they feel they are not getting paid their worth - they will quit and leave behind depleted numbers, thus more workload for you. Therefore, use your voice to stand up for nurses, especially female nurses.

Another way to change negative perceptions female nurses may have towards you is to be a lot more collaborative. While male nurses are fighting gender stereotypes in the nursing field, men also are fighting the view that they always need to be leading or are not masculine enough, especially around women.

So, that masculine urge to show 'leadership' in an all-female unit might lead to a man putting himself in an awkward situation of trying to take over roles that more experienced nurses, most of whom will be women, could easily handle. Perhaps this attitude to wanting to lead regardless of experience or knowledge could make female nurses view male nurses' entry into the field in a negative light. This could be why they might see you less as a colleague and more as a competition.

Therefore, to get nurses to trust you and change any negative perception they may have about male nurses, enter the field with a collaborative mindset. Rather than give in to that urge to just take the leadership role while you are still new there, consider taking the back seat and working with the other nurses to create a positive impression from them about what it means to be a male nurse. Listen to instructions from senior female nurses or doctors, take criticism well and learn from your mistakes.

Now, this does not mean you should simply roll over each time and forget to stand up for yourself. Rather, relate to the female nurses as you would relate to your male colleagues in a professional setting. Be willing to learn from them, follow instructions, and be open to asking questions or suggesting different ways of doing things. Just don't be obnoxious while you do this. That would only perpetuate the negative perception that male nurses are not cut for the nursing profession.

However, no matter what you do, a female nurse changing her perspective will be dependent on her alone at the end of the day. So, the above actions can be suitable catalysts to get people to change how they view male nurses. Still, unfortunately, they are no guarantee that female nurses with negative views of male nurses will change their perception completely.

At some point, female nurses will need to come to terms with their perceptions, and only then will they change. Thus, while you need to give a good impression of who you are at work, the only people who can completely change their negative perception of male nurses in the hospital are female nurses.

With the understanding that nurses are in high demand and in short supply, it will not take long for those against men entering into nursing to realize that we need more nurses regardless of gender and, thus, change how they look at male nurses.

The Pay Gap Issue

The gender pay gap is no doubt one of the most pertinent issues in nursing. Men, a minority in the field, earn higher on average than their female counterparts. Therefore, it is understandable that many female nurses view men's entry into the field as taking away from the profession rather than adding to it.

This is one of the biggest pains that female nurses have when male nurses come into question: a male nurse can earn more (on average) than a female nurse for similar roles. But what can lead to the gender pay gap aside from men taking on more hospital responsibilities and roles?

A survey by Nurse.com found that 43 percent of male nurses, compared to just 34 percent of female nurses, negotiated their salary options with their employers. This often comes down to that confidence in men that we spoke about earlier. Men will often feel a lot more deserving of higher pay, while female nurses will often be more likely to suffer from imposter syndrome, meaning that they feel as though they may not be worthy of higher pay. Thus, the female nurse who feels this way looks at a male nurse's confidence in a negative light, leading to a negative perception of male nurses.

This negative perception is beyond the nurses themselves. Thus, it cannot be overcome by female nurses simply needing to get over it, nor can it be overcome by male nurses simply acting like it doesn't exist.

Female nurses, rather than look at the pay gap as a negative to the nursing profession, can use their male counterparts' higher salaries to demand better pay from their employers. Female nurses have been holding up the healthcare sector for up to a century now and, thus, are much more adapted to modern medicine than male nurses, even though nursing had previously been a field for males only.

Therefore, their presence in the nursing field is necessary. Thus, female nurses must stand up for themselves and demand better pay from their employers, equal to their male counterparts for similar roles, specialties, and education levels.

Turning the gender pay gap against male nurses will do nothing for the female nurse, nor will it do anything for the nursing field. Instead, what will happen is that the two genders will create a toxic work environment for each other, leading to a diminished capacity to care for patients.

Female nurses should also increase their education so that they can obtain better certifications that will put them in a better position to negotiate for higher pay. On the other hand, male nurses should also fight for more pay for female nurses.

Additionally, the more we hire men in nursing, the more we are breaking gender stereotypes and alleviating the nursing shortage across the country. A disregard for gender means that we hire the best and most qualified people for the profession. The qualifications for nursing should be on core characteristics such as empathy, patience, kindness, and personality – level-headed, calm and collected, outgoing – and not be placed on gender.

Because as we know, not all women are empathetic and outgoing, and on the other end, not all men are those things either. But hiring the people who best embody the traits, whether male or female, is the best way to get the best people on the job.

Conclusion

Being a male nurse is becoming more of a norm than we think. Although the numbers are increasing, there is such great potential for them to grow faster than they currently are. Current male nurses are in the perfect position to really inspire young men to venture into the nursing field.

Yes, there are benefits, including flexible working hours and a competitive salary. However, nothing beats knowing that what you did in terms of patient interventions gave them a foundation to achieve better health.

We are not saying that aiding in the progression of the nursing profession will be easy. There are times when male nurses may be stereotyped against. But, by standing firm and meeting these stereotypes with strategized comments that do not insult but rather educate, we are in a way beating this stereotypical system.

As a male nurse, you provide yourself with opportunities many can only dream of. You can choose specialties that best suit your personality while being able to nurture and spend time with your family. It is often said that you cannot have it all; however, no profession other than nursing can provide you with the fulfillment and opportunity to progress as far as you want. Becoming a male nurse is rare, but the impact you are having and the motivation you are providing young men will be evident very far in nursing and the healthcare field as a whole.

As a male nurse, you are unique! You can, and you will excel more than you ever thought possible! Never let anyone ever tell you that you cannot survive the process.

References

All Nurses. (2019, December 6). The Stigma of Men in Nursing. Allnurses. https://allnurses.com/the-stigma-men-nursing-t711858/

Baneas, D. (2021). I'm a Male Nurse and I Choose Nursing. Www.farrerpark.com. https://www.farrerpark.com/medical-professionals/Nursing-Department/Care-Gallery/Im-a-Male-Nurse-and-I-Choose-Nursing.html

Bradley University. (2018, June 15). The Growth of Male Nurses in Health Care | Bradley University Online. Bradley University Online. https://onlinedegrees.bradley.edu/blog/the-growth-of-male-nurses-in-health-care/

Daniels, L. (2013, April 18). Are you a "murse", a "male nurse" or simply a "nurse"? Nursing Times. https://www.nursingtimes.net/students/are-you-a-murse-a-male-nurse-or-simply-a-nurse-18-04-2013/

December 27, C. P. • U., & 2018. (2019, September 3). Wellness Nurse Job Description. Career Trend. https://careertrend.com/about-6544427-wellness-nurse-job-description.html

Demaria, J. (2011, July 4). 3 myths about men in nursing. Scrubs | the Leading Lifestyle Magazine for the Healthcare Community. https://scrubsmag.com/male-nurse-myths/

EveryNurse Staff. (2019). Strategies for Dealing with a Challenging Colleague | EveryNurse.org. EveryNurse. https://everynurse.org/strategies-dealing-with-challenging-colleague/

International Student. (2020). Nursing Programs in the US | Study Nursing in the US. International Student. https://www.internationalstudent.com/study-nursing/nursing-programs-in-the-us/

Jean, J. (2019). The importance of male representation in nursing. Dhge.org. https://dhge.org/about-us/blog/male-representation-in-nursing

Kareplus. (2016, October 6). 4 Famous Male Nurses. Kare plus Head Office. https://kareplus.co.uk/blog/2016/10/06/4-famous-male-nurses/

KidsHealth Medical Experts. (2021). Confidence (for Teens) - Nemours KidsHealth. Kidshealth.org. https://kidshealth.org/en/teens/confidence.html#:~:text=Confidence%20helps%20us%20feel%20ready

Mary. (2016, September 9). 6 Male Nurses in History You Should Know (But Probably Don't) - NurseBuff. NurseBuff. https://www.nursebuff.com/male-nurses-in-history/

Morris, G. (2022, July 21). The Importance Of Male Representation In Nursing | NurseJournal. Nursejournal.org. https://nursejournal.org/articles/male-nursing-representation/

R.N, R. C. (2016, May 4). 3 Myths About Male Nurses You're Probably Tired Of Hearing. Nurseslabs. https://nurseslabs.com/3-myths-male-nurses-youre-probably-tired-hearing/

Slyter, K. (2018, March 12). Men in Nursing Reveal What It's Really Like Working in a Female-Dominated Field | Rasmussen College. Www.rasmussen.edu. https://www.rasmussen.edu/degrees/nursing/blog/men-in-nursing/

Other Books By The Author

Career Exploration Guide: https://www.amazon.com/dp/1734865725

Rich Nurse How to start a Nursing Business: https://www.amazon.com/dp/1734865709

The Real Issue in Nursing Stress and Mental Illness: https://www.amazon.com/dp/B0BFFW4LRY/

Operation Ugly Truth: A Nurse's Firsthand account of the NYC Pandemic: https://www.amazon.com/dp/1734865733

The Journey To Respect starts with You: 7 days Inspirational Black Book: https://mybook.to/RESPECT

The Real Guide to Teenage Depression: Handling Teen Depression: https://mybook.to/Esyqy

The Great Big Slap: Slapping is Unacceptable: https://mybook.to/TheGreatBigSlap

Wish You Knew The Family Wanted Your Love: https://mybook.to/WISHYOUKNEW

Broken Teen Scars: https://mybook.to/BrokenTeenScars

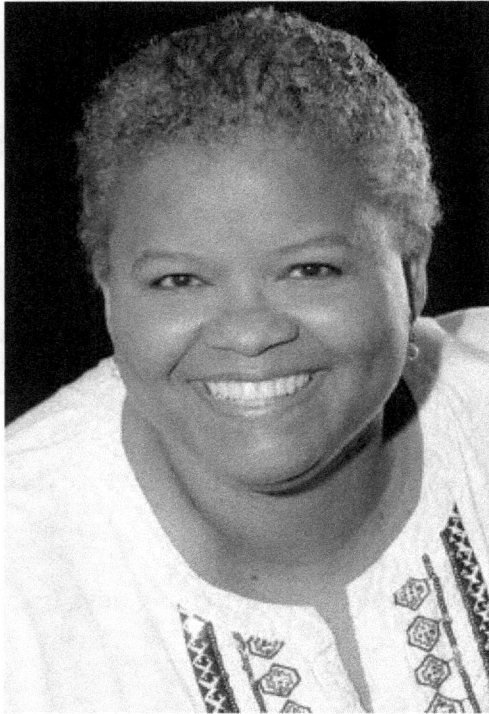

© Patrice M Foster

Learn More About Patrice M. Foster From:

https://patricemfoster.com

www.ingramcontent.com/pod-product-compliance
Lightning Source LLC
Chambersburg PA
CBHW052220270326
41931CB00011B/2419